12 Step Detox

12 Step Detox

Dr. Christopher J. Dorais

ISBN-13: 9781518860676
ISBN-10: 1518860672
Library of Congress Control Number: 2015918237
CreateSpace Independent Publishing Platform
North Charleston, South Carolina

"My people perish for a lack of knowledge."

~HOSEA 4:6

Introduction

n 2001, my health utterly collapsed due to toxicity. The results of this collapse were powerful chemical sensitivities, food allergies, chronic fatigue, depression, memory lapses, crippling back pain, frequent hives and swelling, and a pathetically weak immune system. In short, my body—and my life—was a mess. Back in those days, the word "detox" seemed to be only associated with drug and alcohol abuse. Now we hear about detoxing all of the time, and it usually has nothing to do with drugs or alcohol. How quickly things have changed.

Last year, I wrote my first book, *Detox Memoir*, because I wanted to share the story of my twelve-year journey from sickness to health. Since writing *Detox Memoir*, many people have asked me: "What can I do right now to detox myself?" This is an excellent question, as it gets to the very heart of the matter. Whether we realize it or not, all of us are experiencing health issues of some sort or another due to toxicity. This is because we live in an increasingly toxic world. What can we do to stop, limit, or slow the damage done to our bodies because of the toxins in our food, water, air, and soil? We even produce toxins in our own bodies. How can we protect ourselves from these poisonous substances before they ruin our health?

After more than a decade of researching toxicity and experimenting with detox protocols, I am convinced that the most effective detox protocols do not involve any expensive supplements. Yes, you can breathe that sigh of relief now. This book does not require you to buy super-expensive supplements and go on absurd crash diets for ridiculously long periods of time. Yes, taking supplements and making some dietary changes are important. However, they are not essential to an effective detox program. The reason for this is very simple. The most important part of detoxing is not what you put in your body, but what you take out. A great detox program should not focus on putting exceedingly expensive supplements into your body, but on taking relatively inexpensive chemicals out. Once we clean our body of the toxins it has accumulated over the years, the body is very often fully able to repair itself in the exact manner in which it requires.

When I was 17 years old, I bought my first car. It was a total clunker. Still, I loved that old car, and I wanted to take care of it. My older brother, who was then and is still today, a talented mechanic, gave me some basic, but essential, car maintenance advice. "Make sure you change the oil a few times a year, and be sure to change the oil filter when you change the oil." Anyone who has worked on cars understands the reason for this. In a way, oil is the life blood of the engine. You put that new golden-colored motor oil into the engine, and the car runs great. But, after a few thousand miles of driving, the oil has changed to a dark brown—or even a dirty black. This dark and dirty oil needs to be changed, or it will eventually damage the engine. The oil filter did its job the best that it could, but there comes a point in time when the filter is so dirty that it can no longer clean the oil. So, we replace both filter and oil together in order to properly maintain our engine. Well, we cannot replace the blood in our bodies, nor can we directly clean out the blood—*but we can clean the blood filters*. This is exactly what a good detox does. It cleans the body's filters. All filters get dirty over time. This is why detoxing periodically is essential for great health.

The human body contains several filters. These filters cannot be changed like an oil filter, at least not without surgery. However, these filters can be cleaned. This cleaning should be done on a regular basis. The problem is that most people are very conscientious about changing their car's oil, air, and fuel filters, but never consider cleaning even one of their own biological filters! No wonder health problems are reaching epidemic levels.

As I was struggling to find answers to my own toxicity issues, I began to think that all these new health problems I was experiencing were simply due to aging. *Old age had finally caught up with me and I would just have to adjust to this terrible new normal.* Then I began to think that perhaps this was just some sort of "bad health phase" that I stumbled into, and that it would gradually pass over time. I was wrong on both counts. My health problems were not due to aging, nor did these problems diminish over time. My health problems got progressively worse. This went on for several years. When I finally started making progress with my research and experimentation, I found that these health problems were strangely simple in origin. Several of my biological filters were dirty, just like my old clunker's oil filter. Four of my biological filters—the thyroid, kidneys, liver, and intestines, desperately needed cleaning. They needed their periodic maintenance. However, in my ignorance, I had disregarded their maintenance schedule. Once I began cleaning out these filters, my body was able to repair itself, and my health problems began to vanish.

It took me over five years to learn this basic fact—that my body filters were dirty and needed cleaning. Then it took me another seven years of doctor's visits, research, and trial and error to learn how to clean these filters. The reason it took me so long to do this was that I had almost no idea of what I was doing in those early days of detoxing. I made far more wrong turns than right turns back then. Indeed, there were times when I felt that basically everything I was trying to do to improve my health was wrong.

Eventually I found my way through that dark, miserable forest of sickness and disease. During my journey through that darkness, I kept a journal that I continually updated with my latest research findings. This journal was my road map back to good health, and it became the foundation for this book, *12 Step Detox.*

You may find in the reading of this book that not all of the twelve steps are of equal value to you. This is completely normal. Each person's detox needs may be different because of the large number of variables at work. Some people may need to take only one or two of the twelve steps in order to recover their health. There are variables of frequency of exposure, intensity of exposure, and the duration of exposure to toxins. Also, our genetics play an important factor.

All of these variables make detoxing an extremely complex process. But there is good news in all of this. Chemical toxins share a tremendous amount of common ground with each other. They all have affected the human filtration areas because toxins are collected by the filters. *12 Step Detox* explains how to clean up these filtration areas one by one. Add to this cleaning process some supplements to assist the body in healing itself, and you may find what I did: a powerful improvement in both physical and mental well-being that is amazingly profound, and beautiful.

Dedication

This book is dedicated to anyone who has spent countless hours in hospitals and medical clinics looking for highly elusive answers to perplexing health problems. I was that person many years ago. If this is you, I know all too well the wretched frustration that you feel. The pain, the loneliness, the tremendous waste of time, energy, and money—all of this is almost unbearable. I am here to tell you that there are answers to your health problems, and this book may contain some of those answers. But it is not enough just to know the answers, you have to implement them. Once I actually started doing the *12 Step Detox*, I started to see wonderful changes in my mind and body. In time, I got my life back.

All people are toxic at some level. The only real difference is that some people are taking active steps to reduce their levels of toxicity. You must take an active role in doing this in order to regain your life back. This is my desire, hope, and prayer for you.

Disclaimer

THE CONTENTS OF THIS BOOK ARE FOR EDUCATIONAL AND INFORMATIONAL PURPOSES ONLY. NEITHER THE AUTHOR NOR THE PUBLISHER IS ENGAGED IN RENDERING PROFESSIONAL MEDICAL ADVICE OR MEDICAL SERVICES TO THE READER. THIS BOOK IS NOT MEANT TO BE **MEDICAL ADVICE,** NOR IS IT A **PRESCRIPTION** FOR ANY ILLNESS OR CONDITION. THE AUTHOR AND THE PUBLISHER ARE NOT LIABLE OR RESPONSIBLE FOR ANY LOSS, INJURY, OR DAMAGE ALLEGEDLY ARISING FROM ANY INFORMATION OR SUGGESTION IN THIS BOOK. THE AUTHOR AND THE PUBLISHER ARE ABSOLVED OF ANY RESPONSIBILITY ARISING FROM ANY USE OF THIS INFORMATION.

THESE STATEMENTS ARE TO BE CONSIDERED DISCLAIMERS OF RESPONSIBILITY FOR ANYTHING PUBLISHED HERE. THE AUTHOR AND PUBLISHER PROVIDE THE INFORMATION IN THIS BOOK WITH THE UNDERSTANDING THAT YOU MAY ACT ON IT AT YOUR OWN RISK AND ALSO WITH THE FULL KNOWLEDGE THAT HEALTH PROFESSIONALS SHOULD ALWAYS BE CONSULTED FIRST BEFORE ANY ACTION IS TAKEN. YOU SHOULD FIRST CONSULT WITH A PHYSICIAN WHO IS KNOWLEDGEABLE AND TRAINED IN ALTERNATIVE AND NATURAL HEALING MODALITIES TO DETERMINE WHETHER ANY OF THE PROTOCOLS AND PROCEDURES DISCUSSED IN THIS BOOK WORK, OR WHETHER THEY ARE OF ANY VALUE.

Table of Contents

CHAPTER 1

A History of Toxicity

Every person is toxic. No one is immune to this because we live in a toxic world. Pollutants are all around us, and in us. Certainly there are degrees of toxicity between people. Toxicity differs due to a number of variables (genetics, time, duration of exposure, toxin types) but we are all affected by these toxins. Unfortunately, the effects of toxicity are *always* negative. Getting splashed by toxic waste one day and turning into a superhero the next day only occurs in the virtual world of fantasy. In the real world, the result of toxicity is always bad. Whether it is the common cold or cancer, toxicity affects everyone. How did this get so bad? Usually when people consider this question, they put the blame directly at the feet of heavy industry and their polluting factories. This is misplaced blame. Industrial pollution accounts for only a very small percent of the actual problem. I believe the problem of toxicity is something nearer, much closer to home. It is also more easily controlled. Most of us have little or no influence with what the big factory in town is doing, but we do have influence over ourselves. This is where the real battle is. It starts and ends with us.

None of us were able to choose who our mothers were. This was chosen for us. The same is true for our grandmothers, and great-grandmothers. I don't blame my mother or her mother for my toxicity problems. They didn't know any better. But they were the start of my problems, just the same, and I am not talking about genetics. I am talking about mercury metal.

As long as I can remember, my mother had terrible teeth. She passed away due to liver failure when she was only 70 years old. By time time, nearly every tooth in her mouth had a metal filling of some sort. My mother had mercury fillings at a very young age. It is a proven fact that mercury metal from fillings leaches into a person's body every day. If a person has mercury fillings, every time they swallow, they are ingesting a lethal toxin. Yes, this is only in very small amounts. But over time, this accumulation can become deadly. It is a slow-kill. Mercury will eventually attack every major system in the human body, beginning with the human immune system. While all of this sounds horrible—and it is—the most devastating aspect of mercury is its ability to pass from one generation to the next.

Mercury can do this because it has the incredible ability to pass through both the brain-blood barrier and the fetal-blood barrier. This means that after I was conceived, my little body was built with mercury-tainted blood coming from my mother. After I was born, I was nursed with mercury-laced milk. If my maternal grandmother had mercury fillings (and I could not find anyone in my family who could confirm or deny this), then my mother had also received mercury from her mother. This generational transmission of mercury has affected billions of people on our planet. I imagine right now you would be hard pressed to find even one person whose mother or maternal grandmother did not have mercury (euphemistically known as "silver amalgam") fillings in their mouth. If your mother or grandmother has or had those silvery metal fillings in their mouth, you can be sure you have mercury in your body also. You may be thinking, "if that is true, then just about everyone I know has mercury in their bodies." *Exactly*.

Mercury toxicity is one of the biggest health hazards in the world, and yet few people are talking about it anymore. It is considered passé in most scholarly circles today. The world has moved on with supposedly more important health concerns. Meanwhile, mercury continues on inflicting terrible damage to people of every nation, generation after generation.

What kind of damage can mercury do? *Plenty*. And all of it is bad. Cardiac, respiratory, neurological, musculature, endocrine, reproductive, digestive— you name it, and mercury can damage it. Every major system from head to toe can be affected by mercury. The human body's filters, along with the human immune system, are on the front lines of this toxicity battle. Because a person's entire blood supply passes through this area every hour, probably one of the first recipients of this toxic mercury flowing in your bloodstream is a tiny gland that is increasingly getting people's attention: the thyroid. Mercury is strongly attracted to thyroid gland tissues because these tissues contain very high levels of selenium, an element that mercury has a powerful affinity towards. This is one reason why a thyroid cleanse is an essential part of the *12 Step Detox*. Unfortunately, there is another reason why people's thyroids are failing them at near epidemic levels. Not only does the tiny thyroid get absolutely punished by mercury, it also takes a beating from the second main source of toxicity in our environment: ordinary tap water.

In the United States, the typical municipal water supply is "purified" by two chemicals that directly attack the human thyroid: chlorine and fluorine. These two chemicals, known as halides or halogens, are in the same family as iodine. The thyroid contains the highest concentration of iodine in the human body. It uses iodine molecules to make thyroid hormones, and to boost the body's immune system. Without an adequate supply of iodine, the thyroid suffers, which in turn causes the body to suffer. Chlorine and fluorine are in a very real sense, chemically speaking, related to iodine. They are also more powerful than iodine. When the human body is exposed to chlorine and fluorine, the thyroid will receive these elements at the expense of vital iodine. The body will actually flush iodine out through the urine to receive the chlorine and fluorine. This is a type of poisoning. It is slow, but terribly effective.

Are you now beginning to see why detoxing is so important? Mercury passed through the generations on the one hand, toxic halogens in our tap water on the other. The end result is an entire population that is sick and getting sicker. Clearly, we live in a world that is in desperate need of detoxing.

If this rather depressing information has your head literally swimming, there is good news in all of this. Detoxing can reverse this terrible downward spiral! The tiny thyroid, which is one of the four main filters in the human body, can be cleaned out. It can be "rebooted." You just have to know how to do it. I rebooted my thyroid with incredible results, and I will show you how I did it in a future chapter. However, before we get to that, we need to take our very first step in detoxing. We need to get a "damage report" on ourselves.

DETOX STEP #1: Take a Toxin Inventory.

If we want to measure our progress in a quantitative manner, it is important to get hard data. People may lie or imagine themselves feeling better as time goes on, but numbers neither lie nor do they have an imagination. The first of the 12 detox steps is to obtain baseline data of your present condition. Here are the baseline numbers from my first hair analysis. I chose the hair analysis over blood or urine analysis because I believe the hair shows long term trends of toxicity far more accurately. Besides its accuracy, the hair analysis is convenient, and very cost-effective. All I did was cut off a bit of hair and ship it to a lab (see Appendix) for analysis. After a few weeks, I received a report in the mail, which included this chart.

POTENTIALLY TOXIC ELEMENTS (My Baseline)				
	RESULT µg/g	RANGE	PERCENTILE	
			68th	95th
Aluminum	25.0	< 12.0		
Antimony	0.054	< 0.080		
Arsenic	0.11	< 0.120		
Bismuth	0.040	< 2.0		
Cadmium	0.029	< 0.150		
Lead	0.750	< 2.0		
Mercury	0.30	< 1.10		
Uranium	0.090	< 0.060		
Nickel	1.100	< 0.40		
Silver	0.22	< 0.10		
Tin	0.84	< 0.30		
Titanium	0.78	< 1.00		
Total Toxic Representation				

The phrase "potentially toxic elements" refers to the harmful elements that were in my system at the time of the hair test. The numbers indicate the levels at which they were found in the hair sample. Black lines that reach into the 95th percentile column meant that I was in the extreme range of toxicity. The hair analysis report is actually a statistical and probability report of how your body chemistry compares to everyone else's. If you are in this 95th percentile range, you are in an exclusive class of toxicity, along with the other unfortunate 5 percent of the people who have an extremely high level of a particular toxin. This is bad—very bad.

As you can see from this report, I had extremely high levels of nickel and tin in my system. While this was disturbing, it was not unexpected, because I had been orally ingesting tin and nickel every day for the last twenty years or so. You see, ever since I was very young, I had amalgam metal fillings in my mouth. Every day, a small portion of these fillings were worn away by chewing and saliva. Amalgam metal fillings are just that—an amalgam. This sounds harmless enough until you discover that the amalgam is actually made up of mercury, silver, tin, nickel, copper, and a few other elements. For over twenty years, I had been ingesting toxic metals, two of which are extremely poisonous—mercury and nickel—every minute of every day. *What a depressing situation!*

Besides the amalgam fillings, I also had four root canals. Some root canal materials—particularly with older root canals—contain toxic metals, including a significant amount of nickel. So even from a cursory overview, this first hair analysis report made a great deal of sense to me. The high toxic levels were certainly not what I wanted to see. However, they were exactly what I expected to see, because I had received mercury from my own mouth, and from my mother.

That's enough bad news for now. Let's consider the good news. Effective detoxing can undo much of the damage done by these toxins. When looking over your own hair analysis report, the goal of your detoxing is very clear: shorten the length of those long black lines. You must reduce the sizes of the numbers in the RESULT column. Ideally, you don't want even one element to be in the middle 68th to 95th percentile range. I had five elements in my baseline data that reached into this dangerous range, with one element—nickel—past the 95th percentile.

Everyone's goal in detoxing is the same: get into the lowest range of these elements. If possible, you want to get to a point where you do not even have a line on this chart at all.

If you look at the bottom of my baseline data, you will see a summative line entitled "Total Toxic Representation." I estimate I came in around the 75th percentile in terms of a total toxic representation. From a sheer statistical and probability point of view, I was sicker than approximately 74 percent of the other people who have taken a hair analysis, or at least this is how I looked at it. Many people don't like hair analysis specifically because it deals with statistics and probability. But for my part, the hair analysis suited my purposes perfectly. I wanted baseline data, and now I had it. I had a summative measurement in the total toxic representation number, and I had real quantitative data concerning various dangerous elements that were currently in my body. Most conveniently, I had done this all from the comfort of my own home.

POTENTIALLY TOXIC ELEMENTS (at 17 months)				
	RESULT µg/g	RANGE	PERCENTILE	
			68th	95th
Aluminum	14.0	<12.0		
Antimony	0.035	<0.080		
Arsenic	0.11	<0.120		
Bismuth	0.047	<2.0		
Cadmium	0.038	<0.150		
Lead	0.52	<2.0		
Mercury	0.07	<1.10		
Uranium	0.11	<0.060		
Nickel	0.26	<0.40		
Silver	0.02	<0.10		
Tin	0.38	<0.30		
Titanium	0.52	<1.00		
Total Toxic Representation				

Toxin	Original Level	After 17 Months	% Increase or Decrease
Aluminum	25.0	14.0	44% Decrease
Antimony	0.054	0.035	35% Decrease
Arsenic	0.11	0.11	No Change
Bismuth	0.040	0.047	18% Increase
Cadmium	0.029	0.038	31% Increase
Lead	0.750	0.52	31% Decrease
Mercury	0.30	0.07	77% Decrease
Uranium	0.090	0.11	222% Increase
Nickel	1.10	0.26	76% Decrease
Silver	0.22	0.02	91% Decrease
Tin	0.84	0.38	55% Decrease
Titanium	0.78	0.52	33% Decrease

After 17 months of detoxing, I sent the lab another hair sample for analysis and I received the results shown here. The improvements were encouraging when compared against the baseline data, and this was only after detoxing for 17 months. And much of this detoxing was done the wrong way because I still had so much to learn concerning the proper way to detox.

Still, I felt so much better now than before I began my detox. However, just *feeling* better wasn't good enough. I needed hard data to back up these feelings. With this second hair analysis report, I had that data. Looking at numbers from a different perspective, I found that of the twelve toxic elements tested in the hair analysis, I had a significant reduction in eight of these. When I combined all of the numbers in the "% Increase or Decrease" column and divided by 12, I found that I had decreased my overall toxic burden by 14.25%. And this was done by a detox novice who, in his early days, made far more wrong turns than right. If I could have done this all over again—had I known detoxing should be done according to a sequence of twelve logical steps—I am certain this number would have been significantly higher after 17 months.

26 months into my detox journey, I sent in yet another hair sample. Here is the raw data taken from that report.

Toxin	Original Level	After 26 Months	% Increase or Decrease
Aluminum	25.0	9.3	63% Decrease
Antimony	0.054	0.017	69% Decrease
Arsenic	0.11	0.11	No Change
Bismuth	0.040	0.050	25% Increase
Cadmium	0.029	0.014	52% Decrease
Lead	0.750	0.27	64% Decrease
Mercury	0.30	<0.03	90% Decrease
Uranium	0.090	0.26	188% Increase
Nickel	1.10	0.10	91% Decrease
Silver	0.22	<0.006	97% Decrease
Tin	0.84	0.05	94% Decrease
Titanium	0.78	0.30	62% Decrease

At this point, I was experiencing some truly impressive gains and I was feeling so much better. Adding all of the percentages in the far right column and dividing by 12, I found that I reduced my toxic burden from my baseline by an incredible 39%. Sure, the numbers looked great, but the important thing was the numbers matched how I felt. The numbers looked great, and I felt great!

REVIEW OF DETOX STEP #1: Take a Toxin Inventory

Get an analysis to find your baseline levels of toxicity. I recommend a hair analysis because it shows long term trends, which neither blood nor urine are able to show. Also, the hair analysis is both convenient and cost-effective. As you detox, you will want to get a second, third, and even fourth toxin inventory. As you begin to see and feel certain improvements in your condition, future toxicity reports will provide both encouragement and direction to your detox efforts as you move forward.

TIME/DURATION: This inventory should be taken before any detox protocols are started in order to accurately assess the initial body burden of toxicity. This can be repeated every six months thereafter to evaluate the progress of your detoxing efforts.

CHAPTER 2

Stopping the Source

After taking a toxin inventory to see where you rank in terms of your own toxicity, the next best step is to stop the inflow of new toxins entering your body—if you can. It doesn't make much sense to detox if you continually expose yourself to new toxins. This is like trying to fill a bathtub without first plugging the drain. Yes, doing a good detox will give you positive results whether you stop the flow of incoming toxins or not. However, when you cut the supply line of the current toxin influx, you can turn a good detox strategy into a great one. Stopping the inflow of toxins gives the body a much-needed rest from the toxic battle it is waging. Instead of using its resources to fight a war, the body can now utilize its resources for rebuilding and recovery. If you want quick healing, you must stop doing what is hurting you.

DETOX STEP #2: Cut the Toxic Supply Line.

It took a great deal of research before I became thoroughly convinced that my own metal fillings were one of the main sources of my health problems. I also struggled with the idea that the heavily chlorinated and fluoridated water that I was drinking and washing with on a daily basis was also hurting my health. I read both sides of the argument. One group says that mercury fillings are mostly inert. This was essentially the same group that said the trace levels of chlorine and fluorine in the municipal water supply were safe. The other side said exactly the opposite, that mercury, chlorine, and fluorine are responsible for a huge number of health problems worldwide, and should be avoided at all costs. *Which side was I to believe?* Instead of focusing on what these two opposing sides disagreed on, I focused on what they agreed upon. Both stated that these elements were dangerous poisons. *Dangerous poisons. Why should I expose my body, which was already spiraling downward in health, to even one molecule of a poison?* I spent countless hours doing the research, but when it came time to make a truly safe choice, it was actually a very easy one to make. The mercury, chlorine, and fluorine were all supply lines for toxicity. If I was going to recover my health, this inflow had to stop. Trace amounts meant that the poisons were still there, so these supply lines had to be cut.

Even if cutting a toxic supply line is an easy decision to make—I mean, who wouldn't want to *stop* ingesting poison—it can be difficult to implement. We know we need to do something, but we don't often want to do it. Part of the reason for this is that by taking this sort of action, we directly contradict what many supposed experts in their fields have said and done. Mercury, fluorine, and chlorine are highly toxic substances. These toxins were put into our bodies and into our water supply by professionals. These are people we should be able to trust. *They wouldn't do this if they knew that this actually harms people, would they?* That's a good question for which I do not have an answer. I couldn't answer the question of the motives of these so-called experts. Then again, I didn't really need to. People may lie, but numbers never do. Neither do chemicals. A poison is a poison.

With regards to mercury amalgam fillings, I had accumulated research over the course of several years from the U.S. Food and Drug Administration, the American Dental Association, the American Medical Association, and the World Health Organization on the dangers of mercury. There was just too much scholarly research to ignore. Yes, some of these organizations discounted the dangers of the small amounts of mercury leaching from fillings on a daily basis. But I didn't discount these amounts. When only one atom of this toxic metal can potentially deactivate an entire living cell, it was clear to me that there was no such thing as a safe amount of mercury. My mercury fillings were slowly poisoning me on a daily basis. The only logical decision was to cut this supply line of toxicity. It was clear the mercury fillings had to go.

I made an appointment with a local biological dentist (a person specifically trained to remove mercury fillings), and had all six of my fillings removed. While this was very good progress towards cutting my toxic supply line, I found another source of mercury that I was inadvertently exposing myself to. This source had to be eliminated as well.

Back in 2009, the Washington Post broke a story on how traces of mercury were found in high fructose corn syrup (HFCS). Many people know that mercury is very frequently found in fish, and in vaccinations in a form called *thimerosal*. All this was horrible enough—and now mercury is in our cereals, sodas, jellies, and bread? *No wonder so many people are sick these days!* All the food in my pantry that contained HFCS, and it was no small amount, went into the trash. I already had enough mercury in my system from my mother and from my own fillings. I didn't need to add more of this toxic metal into my already over-burdened body as a result of eating a peanut butter and jelly sandwich with the wrong kinds of bread and jelly.

With the mercury supply line now cut, I focused my attention on another significant source of toxicity, the chlorine and fluorine in my tap water. I was particularly interested in getting rid of the fluorine because I found that fluorine actually has the ability to amplify the destructive capabilities of other toxins in the body—including mercury. My thyroid was never going to get better if I continually drank and bathed in water that contained two chemicals—fluorine and chlorine—that specifically cause my body to excrete iodine. I needed that iodine!

The thyroid requires huge amounts of iodine to make thyroid hormones. Iodine also provides a big boost to the human immune system. On the other hand, iodine deficiency has a very strong correlation with a great many types of diseases, including several types of cancer—breast, prostate, and thyroid just to name a few. After a great deal of research, I began to see anything that specifically targeted the body's precious iodine supply as a serious threat to anyone's health.

This being the case, it was now clear that ordinary tap water was a slow but constant threat because of its high fluorine and chlorine content. *The content was so high that I could even smell the chlorine in the tap water.* This was not good. Something had to give here, and I was determined it wasn't going to be my thyroid. So, after some research, I had a moderately priced whole house water purification system installed in our home. This system removed all of the chlorine, much of the fluorine, and a whole host of other chemical undesirables from the tap water. A friend of mine told me that I would see and feel a big difference in how my skin looked and felt after just a few days of showering in non-chlorinated, non-fluoridated water. I have to confess I was skeptical of my friend's claims. *My skin is going to feel softer and smoother after just a few showers? I don't think so.*

It turns out I was wrong about this. My friend was correct. There was indeed a noticeable improvement in my skin tone and texture after just a few days of using the new system. This was an unexpected but welcome surprise.

Besides the mercury fillings, and tap water, there is another significant source of toxicity that needed to be addressed. This source of toxicity was organic—and living. This source also proved to be much more difficult to get rid of than comparatively simple toxins like mercury, fluorine, or chlorine. I actually found cleaning up three of the four human filters—the liver, kidneys, and thyroid—to be relatively easy. For these three areas, it was pretty much just a matter of using the right protocols and supplements. I found cleaning up the intestines to be far more of a challenge. The reason: when the intestines get sick and damaged, they begin to harbor living pathogenic parasites.

Mercury, fluorine, and chlorine are just elements. They don't technically *respond* to a detox protocol. Parasites are different. They are alive. They have been around as long as man has for a reason. Parasites specialize in evading detection, and they will put up a very good fight to remain in the damp, dark places of their world. One good example of this is *Candida albicans*. Candida is a yeast that is found in everyone, and actually provides some services to the human body. When the body's immune system weakens, particularly in the intestinal region, this yeast may transform into a parasitic fungi. Once in a fungal form, the Candida leaves the intestines and can reach into virtually any area of the body. If it can find food, especially sugar, the Candida will feed and grow. There are two problems with this. One, the body needs that food for its own maintenance and growth. The body certainly does not need billions of fungal mouths to feed. Secondly, the waste products of parasites like Candida are toxic to humans. Carbon monoxide, ethanol, ammonia, and perhaps the worst waste product of all, acetaldehyde, are all produced by the Candida fungus. I couldn't prove it, but it was a good bet that these chemicals were behind many of my crippling health problems. These poisons were doing to me what poisons always do: damage or kill living cells. So, I began to address these problems with a series of fairly easy protocols that eventually comprised my Intestinal Cleanse. This cleanse will be discussed in detail in a future chapter.

I felt I was making great progress with eliminating the various sources of toxicity that had damaged my body for decades. However, there was one final source of toxins that I needed to address. These were the surgical implants that had been placed in my body several years earlier. The dangers of surgical implants is a popular topic of debate, and frankly, it is one that is much bigger than what can be fully examined in this chapter. I had four dental implants. These were all in the form of root canals, and I wanted all of them removed. Of course, there are other types of implants as well. Some of these by their very nature, such as a bone brace, are implants that cannot be removed. Other implants are cosmetic in nature. These *can* be removed. I believe the main problem with all implants is very similar to the fungal parasite issue. Any man-made substance that is placed into a human body will be attacked by resources within the body. For example, bacteria and fungi will attack a dental implant. Nothing can stop this. This is what these microorganisms were designed to do. They attack and break substances down into simpler chemicals. To pretend that these parasites will not attack a dental, breast, or any other type of man-made implant is foolhardy. The fungi and bacteria are simply doing their job. But again, the problem is these microorganisms excrete metabolic wastes that are toxic to humans. Many people argue about the dangers of breast implants from the perspective that if, or when, the implant leaks, a tremendous amount of damage will result. I think this aspect of an implant's danger is too obvious even to discuss. *Of course a leaky implant is dangerous!*

The real problem with implants is much more subtle. It is the fungi, bacteria, and even mold that grows around or in an implant that is the real health hazard to people. Fungi, bacteria, and mold will attack and attempt to break down these foreign, non-biological, inorganic substances. This is what an implant is—a foreign, inorganic substance. As that fungus, bacteria, and mold works away on the implant, it excretes metabolic wastes that are toxic to humans. This is the real danger of implants. This is the reason I had my four root canal implants removed.

REVIEW OF DETOX STEP #2: Cut the Toxic Supply Line

Getting those old mercury fillings or root canals removed is best done by a professional that has been specifically trained for this purpose. I used a Biological Dentist for this and this highly skilled professional did an amazing job. All of my metal fillings were removed over a nine month period. My four root canal implants were removed soon after that.

With regards to water filtration systems, there are many good systems available. Of course, those systems that remove more contaminants but retain the good minerals in the water also cost a great deal more. Regardless of the high or low cost of your system, removing as much chlorine and fluorine as possible is paramount. Even if you begin small and simply purchase one filter for a single shower unit, you have made progress in the right direction.

Finally, having a surgical procedure to undo an implant is serious business. If you are in this unfortunate category of people, as I was, I strongly encourage you to do your research. Consider carefully the benefits versus the risks. For some people who are already living on the edge of failing health, there is not much of a decision here. It's either you or your implant. For others who currently appear to be unaffected by the man-made implant, removal is a more delicate decision. You are being affected by the fungi, bacteria, and mold that are attacking your implant, you just are not aware of it at this point. Be sure of this: your immune system is aware of it. Again, all people with implants need to do their homework on this. Look to the research, read the testimonials, and then act accordingly.

TIME/DURATION: Cutting a toxic supply line into your body is actually not essential for detoxing, but it does relieve the body of an enormous toxic burden it is carrying. These lines can be cut before, during, or after your own detox. It is recommended that these lines be cut at the onset of your detox. In this way you will maximize the power of the detox protocols, which could shorten the overall time and energy required to complete your detox.

CHAPTER 3

The Quickest Cleanse

The first detox protocol that a person should do is also the quickest and easiest one to do. The four main detox cleanses (kidney, thyroid, liver, and intestinal) focus on the four main filtration systems of the body. I have three reasons for putting the kidney cleanse at the top of this list for cleanses. First, it's the easiest one to do. This will give anyone confidence who is a bit nervous about doing a detox cleanse. Second, I have found that the kidney cleanse shows powerful results in less than 24 hours. I struggled with lower back pain, particularly in the morning, for many years. Once I discovered the kidney cleanse, I found that my stiff and often aching lower back was vastly improved after just a few cleanses. An effective kidney cleanse clears away debris from the kidneys very quickly. This debris is often a major contributing source of lower back pain and discomfort.

The third reason for doing the kidney cleanse first is because the kidneys produce a large amount of waste on a daily basis. As a person detoxes, the channels for waste elimination must be kept open—wide open. By its very nature, a detox releases a great deal of stored toxins that were formerly trapped within the body. The kidneys should be free and clear of stones and any other sort of residual waste in order to properly manage this increased level of "toxic dumping" that the body will do when a person detoxes.

The kidneys are powerful and effective filters of the human blood. As with all filters, the kidneys collect waste matter, and require periodic cleaning. Yes, the kidneys clean themselves just as all of the body's filters can do. But if the toxin overload is too much for the kidneys, their ability to self-clean declines. In a weakened state, waste matter collects within the kidneys. Many of the substances that tend to collect in the kidneys have the chemical ability to crystalize over time. As the waste matter continues to collect, these tiny crystals grow and become what is known as *kidney stones*. Most people know or have heard that kidney stones are painful, and they are. However, I do not believe that kidney stones alone are to blame for the lower back pain. There is more at work here. As the kidney stones grow, they irritate and inflame the kidney. Inflammation leads to swelling. The now enlarged kidneys press on everything else in the lower back region, including the spine and lower discs, and this can cause stiffness and pain. If you can clean out the kidneys, the irritation is removed, causing the inflammation to be reduced. This in turn, reduces the swelling and the overall size of the kidneys, reducing or even removing the pain.

Because so much waste flows through the urine, kidney cleanses are the logical first step in most detox regimens. They are fast, easy, and effective. Not only should these be done first, they should be done throughout prolonged detoxes. Early on in my detoxing, I found that doing a kidney cleanse every month or so was extremely beneficial. The cleanse keeps the kidney filters clear of obstruction, which allows the other cleanses to work with a far greater efficiency than what they could do otherwise.

DETOX STEP #3: The Kidney Cleanse

Do this first: Buy 12 to 16 lemons, a bunch of parsley, and a packet of asparagus (about 12 to 16 stalks). Try to get all organic produce if possible. You can do this cleanse anytime during the day, but it should be done on an empty stomach. Squeeze 3 or 4 lemons and mix with at least a half-liter of filtered water. Drink within 15 minutes. If you can manage it, repeat this 3 more times until you have consumed 2+ liters of lemon-water. You should try to do this in under two hours.

Do this second: Cut up a handful of parsley into inch-sized pieces and boil in 1-2 cups of filtered water using a glass (Pyrex, etc.) container for about 6-8 minutes. Compress the parsley as it boils, like you are mashing potatoes. This action forces the parsley's essential oils out into the water. Strain out the leaves and stalks and let it cool. You may add ice to speed up the cooling process. Drink the parsley juice. You can mix it with the lemon juice if you like. The taste is not something you will rave about, but it is very possible you will rave about the results of this cleanse.

Do this third: Dice up all of the asparagus stalks into inch-sized pieces like the parsley. Set aside the bottom quarter of these stalks as they are usually too fibrous and tough to eat. Do not cook these. Take the good portions of the asparagus and quick steam them in a glass container for about 5 minutes. Add sea salt, garlic, or even fresh honey to taste. Eat alone or with cooked rice. Some people can eat their asparagus right after drinking their lemon water and "parsley tea." For others, this is just too much food in the stomach too fast. Eat it when you are ready, but do it on the same day as the first two steps.

Assess what you have done: That wasn't so hard was it? All you did was eat a few specific types of food and drink a great deal of purified water. The rest is up to your kidneys! You'll urinate frequently for the next several hours and the smell of your urine may be very pungent. This is the smell of your kidneys being detoxed!

Why this works: The interior of the kidneys look and act like extremely fine filters. These filters are exceedingly sensitive. Anyone who has had kidneys stones understands this. There are at least five different types of crystalline kidney stones. Lemons are strongly acidic and their acids can break up certain types of these hard kidney stones. You drank a great deal of this acid in a short period of time, so your kidneys are flooded with acids that dissolve those painful stones. The asparagus works in a

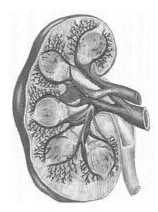

comparable, but opposite way. Asparagus is part of the onion and garlic family, and it contains chemicals that are strongly alkaline. These alkaline substances can also dissolve certain types of stones. Furthermore, the chemicals in the asparagus contain powerful diuretics that make you urinate very frequently. The parsley is similar to the asparagus. It also contains stone-dissolving substances and it is also a strong diuretic. These basic foods contain chemicals which dissolve kidney stones and increase urine production, which causes toxins to be removed quickly from the body.

REVIEW OF DETOX STEP #3: The Kidney Cleanse

There are many kinds of kidney cleanses available. I have used the lemon/parsley/asparagus cleanse numerous times with great success. I still use it today in order to maintain clean kidneys. The main reason for this cleanse is to clear one of the most important excretion pathways of the body. Kidneys work nonstop, and typically produce over a liter of urine a day. They work very hard at keeping the toxins flowing out of your body, so it only makes sense to take care of these two vital filter organs. Clean and clear kidneys allow all of the other detox protocols to proceed much more smoothly, which is why cleaning the kidneys first is a great start to a whole-body detox. Furthermore, cleaning out the kidneys can relieve your lower back of inflammation, which reduces pressure and pain in this very important region of your body.

TIME/DURATION: I recommend doing the kidney cleanse first, and then doing follow-up cleanses about once per month throughout the time of your detoxing. The kidney cleanse is so effective—and so easy to do—it's hard to find any reason not to do it. Of course, if your needs are more severe, you may consider doing this cleanse more frequently.

CHAPTER 4

The Misunderstood Cleanse

O f the four filter cleanses, the kidney cleanse is the easiest to do and the one that shows the fastest results. The second of the four cleanses is also very easy to do, but it takes the longest time to show results. This cleanse is also the most misunderstood cleanse. There are many reasons why the thyroid cleanse is so misunderstood. A big part of this misunderstanding has to do with conventional medical knowledge and treatment concerning the thyroid, and its various disorders. If you do a web search with the words "thyroid" and "misdiagnosis" you will see for yourself how pervasive a problem this misunderstanding is. Clearly there is neither full understanding nor agreement on how the thyroid functions. While there is a great deal of research that still needs to be done concerning this vital gland, here are some basic facts concerning the thyroid that may help your own understanding of this small but exceptionally powerful gland.

Located in the throat and having a mass of only about 30 grams, the thyroid gland is a lightweight in terms of its physical mass. However, because of what it can do, the thyroid in a heavyweight class all by itself. The thyroid produces three hormones, T3 (triiodothyronine), T4 (thyroxine), and calcitonin. The T3 and T4 thyroid hormones influence oxygen consumption and protein production. Put simply, these two hormones control metabolism. Yes, the tiny thyroid produces two substances that affect literally *every* major function in the body because these two hormones influence every cell in the body.

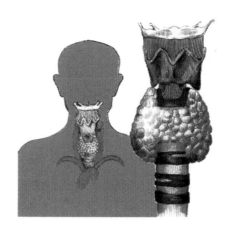

Like all hormones, thyroid hormones are exceedingly powerful. This is probably why the body does not produce the T3 and T4 thyroid hormones in equal amounts. 97% of these two hormones that the thyroid makes is T4. The remaining 3% is T3. Why this disparity? T3 is *five times* more biologically active than T4, and the body simply doesn't need that much metabolism-boosting substance in the blood at one time. When the body does need a metabolic boost, T4 is quickly converted into T3, and the body is ready for action.

This simple conversion is probably the main reason why thyroid function is so difficult to assess. A doctor may conduct a thyroid test and find that it is functioning perfectly, while at the same time the patient still suffers from severe thyroid hormone problems. The problem may not be in the actual thyroid, but in the *conversion* of T4 to T3. If a person is not getting enough thyroid hormone, (hypothyroidism), symptoms like hair loss, weight gain, constipation, slow metabolism, arthritis, fatigue, brain fog, infertility, and dry skin are commonly seen. When a person is getting too much thyroid hormone, (hyperthyroidism), hair loss, infertility, frequent bowel movements, difficulty in keeping normal body weight, irritability, and sleeping disorders are frequently evidenced.

The main point to keep in mind is that this conversion of T4 to T3 occurs in *more places* than just the thyroid. Large quantities of the powerful T3 are generated in the liver, intestines, and even in the kidneys. *Now are you beginning to see why detoxing these filter areas is so important?* You can actually boost your metabolism, and give your thyroid the credit for this boost, when you detox your liver, intestines, or kidneys! This is also why it is very common to pass a thyroid test and yet still suffer from thyroid hormone imbalances. The problem is often somewhere else in the body.

As powerful and important as the thyroid is, it is also extremely sensitive to toxins. Because the entire human blood supply passes through the thyroid gland every hour, the thyroid is particularly vulnerable to toxins that are transported in the blood. This is especially true with certain toxins like mercury, which has a chemical affinity for thyroid gland tissues. Mercury is attracted to the thyroid gland because thyroid tissues contain extremely high amounts of the element selenium, an element which mercury has a powerful affinity towards. This affinity causes mercury that is flowing in the bloodstream to actually be filtered out by the thyroid. These mercury atoms attach to the thyroid, and greatly weaken its ability to function properly. Unfortunately, this may occur very early in life—even before a person is born—because mercury has the unique ability to circumvent the fetal blood barrier. If the mother has mercury issues, she will pass on some of her mercury to her baby's developing thyroid as early as four weeks from conception.

If you think of your thyroid as a filter, you can understand why the thyroid requires periodic cleaning—because all filters require cleaning! Here is an easy protocol you can do with ordinary supplements that has brought slow, but powerful relief to many people with thyroid disorders.

DETOX STEP #4: The Thyroid Cleanse

Do this first: Buy a high quality multivitamin that contains A-E vitamins, including several of the B complex vitamins (B2 and B3 in particular). Make sure this multivitamin contains magnesium as well. Magnesium, B2, and B3 do not directly help the thyroid, but they do assist in the uptake of the three elements the thyroid cleanse absolutely requires: selenium (200 mcg), zinc (40 mg), and iodine. Make sure that you have in your high quality multivitamin zinc, selenium, and magnesium in *chelated* form. If these minerals are not found in your multivitamin in chelated form, then you need to take them in addition to your multivitamin. Chelated minerals are those that are bound to an amino acid.

This allows for greater absorption by the body because when attached to an amino acid, the body recognizes the raw mineral as food.

For selenium, the chelated *selenomethionine* is fantastic. Yet even in chelated form, many elements require absorption assistance. For example, selenium absorption is tied to the presence of Vitamin E. This is one reason why taking a high quality multivitamin is so essential. High quality vitamins tend to have a large variety of "helper vitamins" like Vitamin E, which provide absorption assistance. With the necessary assistance provided, an overall higher level of absorption level is reached. Without good absorption, you are just wasting your money on supplements. The nutrients you think you are absorbing are literally going down the toilet.

Do this second: Buy an iodine supplement. Lugal's 2% and 5% iodine has been a useful iodine supplement for over 150 years, and since it is in liquid form, it is very easy to use. However, some people cannot tolerate the taste and prefer *Iodoral*, which is essentially Lugal's formula in pill form. In either case, the main point is to get iodine into your system. Iodine is the absolute centerpiece of the thyroid cleanse, and the thyroid cleanse is the absolute centerpiece of detoxing. The ultimate success of most of the other detox protocols hinges on thyroid hormones, and these hormones are strongly iodine-dependent.

Iodine is a potent antiseptic, an extremely powerful detoxifying element and cancer-fighting agent, and it is required by every cell in the human body. Not surprisingly, the thyroid gland contains the human body's *greatest* concentration of iodine, with the breasts (in women) and the prostate (in men) also requiring extremely high amounts. Iodine atoms are the most important elements in the T3 and T4 thyroid hormones. Incidentally, this is where the names of these hormones come from. T3 means that triiodothyronine has 3 iodine atoms per molecule, while T4, or thyroxin, has four atoms of iodine per molecule. Without iodine supplementation, the thyroid cleanse will not work.

Do this third: Now that you have all of your needed supplements, you are ready to begin. Start by taking the multivitamin, magnesium, zinc, and selenium supplements for two weeks to prepare your body for the increased levels of iodine it will be receiving. You will probably see your urine become extremely yellow for a time. This is completely normal. It takes a great deal of time for your body to adjust to this new and higher level of nutrient uptake. After about two weeks in this preparatory phase, begin adding iodine to your supplement regimen. Start with only a single drop of Lugal's. If you are using the 2% solution, one drop contains approximately 2.5 mg of iodine. If you are keeping a record of your cleanse, and it is strongly recommended that you do, call this first day of taking your iodine "Day #1." Every 7 days, increase the amount of iodine you take by only one drop. By the end of your first month, you will be taking 4 drops, or 10 mg of iodine per day. At the end of five weeks, the amount will be 12.5 mg of iodine. Many researchers feel that at this level, the body will begin to excrete toxins, including mercury, fluorine, and bromine. If at this point, you just cannot tolerate the taste of Lugal's any longer, you may switch to Iodoral. One pill of Iodoral is the 5-drop equivalent of Lugal's 2%, which is 12.5 mg of iodine. Continue gradually boosting your iodine intake for six months. *Yes, 6 months.* If you feel at any time a "pushback" from your body, reduce your iodine intake temporarily. Going "low and slow" with the supplements, particularly iodine, is vital.

Do this fourth: Now if you have kept to the normal schedule, at the end of six months, you will be taking 24 drops of iodine per day, which is approximately 60 mg per day. Now it is time to "go backwards." Begin dosing down on your iodine by decreasing one drop per week. Keep your other supplements at their normal levels. Continue dosing down until you reach about 5 drops per day (12.5mg). This is considered by many to be an excellent maintenance dosage of iodine.

Assess what you have done: Increasing your iodine levels to higher, but very safe levels, literally pushes the toxic halogens (fluorine, chlorine, and bromine) out of the body. All of this takes time. Not only is iodine required by every cell in the body, there is also a great deal of pushing out of toxic halogens that needs to occur. Furthermore, replenishing vastly depleted storage centers of iodine (in the breasts and the prostate) also takes time. Lastly, iodine assists in the detoxification of mercury, but again, this takes time. Taking your daily iodine doses in gradually increasing amounts greatly minimizes any type of adverse reaction, or "healing crisis" that may occur. Also, doing periodic kidney cleanses and taking your daily iodine in divided doses throughout the day may also ease any discomfort that can occur. After about six or seven months on the thyroid cleanse, you should begin to see some very interesting changes in your body—all of which are good. Reports of having more energy, requiring less sleep, having a better appetite, a stronger immune system, loss of weight, higher metabolism are all commonly reported. Some people even claim to feel vastly younger. This was certainly my personal experience. These are all excellent signs that your thyroid has been cleansed and rebooted.

Why this works: The thyroid is one of the human body's most powerful glands. It also acts as a strong filtering mechanism because the thyroid is exceedingly sensitive to four elements that are extremely common in our environment: mercury (prenatal sources, leaching off of dental fillings), chlorine and fluoride (in most tap water sources), and bromine (found in many types of bread). Chlorine, fluorine, and bromine are all in the same chemical family as iodine. Because they are so closely related chemically, the human body will accept the chlorine, fluorine, and bromine even though they are all toxic. Worse yet, by accepting these toxins, the human body actually has to expel its own iodine. This is one reason why iodine deficiency is so common worldwide. Fortunately, by gradually increasing iodine intake to higher than normal levels for a short period of time, the body can use the iodine to reverse this trend. These high levels allow the body to purge itself of the toxic halogens, as well as the mercury. By slowly reducing the iodine level to a conservative maintenance dosage of around 12.5 mg keeps the thyroid in prime condition, and allows for the body's immune system to enjoy a vast number of protective services (including cancer prevention) that an abundant iodine supply provides.

REVIEW OF DETOX STEP #4: The Thyroid Cleanse

Iodine deficiency is a world-wide problem because toxicity is a world-wide problem. Much of this toxicity targets the tiny and vulnerable thyroid, and its valuable iodine supply. The solution to cleaning up the misunderstood thyroid is a very easy cleanse, but it is not a quick fix. Iodine is a potent element. An extremely powerful anti-cancer agent like iodine has to be powerful in order to be effective. Gradually "dosing up" on your iodine requires a great deal of time, and a generous supply of helper supplements. At the top of the list are high quality forms of selenium, zinc, and magnesium. These elements, along with a high quality multivitamin, work in conjunction with iodine to reboot the tiny but essential thyroid. As you do this your immune system will be significantly boosted and your sluggish metabolism should awaken. Then you may slowly begin to feel different, in a very wonderful way.

TIME/DURATION: It took me over a year of iodine supplementation to re-boot my thyroid, but it was well worth it. The thyroid cleanse can be done concurrently with the other cleanses, so this is one way to save time. However, the thyroid cleanse is a slow cleanse, and my experience in trying to rush it by increasing the iodine dosages too quickly never worked out well. A six month minimum of "dosing up" time is highly recommended, followed by a dosing down time until a 12.5 mg per day maintenance dosage is achieved.

CHAPTER 5

The Dreaded Liver Flush

The liver flush is the third of the four human filter cleanses. The liver flush is undoubtedly the one cleanse that most people find repulsive. If you have ever done a liver flush, more politely known as the *liver cleanse*, you know what I mean. The main reason so many people find the liver flush revolting is not because of what the flush does for a person, but *how* it does it. An effective liver flush will cleanse the liver of obstructions that may have been stuck in a person's body for years. To be rid of this old, useless organic material—clinically known as *gallstones*—is something that most people want. The problem is that most people do not want to do a liver flush to get rid of these stones.

One of the reasons why we feel this way is because gallstones are released in the same manner that regular solid human waste is released. This is true even though gallstones do not look like standard solid waste. Typically, gallstones have a bright greenish tint to them and they float on the surface of the water. This "other-worldly" appearance of gallstones, coupled with the fact that this is old waste matter that came out of a person's rectum probably explains the reason why so many people are disgusted with the liver flush. However, if we can put all aesthetics and real (or feigned) propriety aside for just a short while, we will see the tremendous health-recovering benefits that only a liver flush can provide.

What exactly is a liver flush? Unlike the kidney or thyroid cleanse, the liver flush is not a chemical cleanse at all. It is more of a physical push. It involves very little chemistry and a great deal of physics. As the human body's largest internal organ, the liver carries out a multitude of functions. One of its most important tasks is to assist in keeping the body clean and clear of toxins. As a person's toxin influx increases, the liver's ability to neutralize these toxins decreases. One highly unfortunate consequence of a liver compromised by toxins is that its ability to generate bile is damaged. A healthy adult liver produces about a half liter of liquid bile a day. Bile, which is made up of water, bile salts, cholesterol, and a few other constituents, supports the body both in digestion and detoxification. Bile also assists in the proper use of cholesterol.

We hear a great deal about cholesterol problems today, and we hear a great deal about the ultimate consequence of cholesterol problems—heart disease. What we do not hear nearly enough about is a critical intermediate step in this health-degrading process, which is a compromised liver. When the liver becomes sick due to toxicity, it cannot generate enough high quality bile. This bile shortage weakens the body's detoxification abilities. It also degrades the liver's ability to properly process fats, including cholesterol. Instead, a sick liver will produce an inferior quality and quantity of bile. A sick liver will also produce gallstones. *Yes...gallstones*. These stones are comprised mostly of bile salts and cholesterol, which essentially makes them a coagulated, hardened form of bile. Gallstones originate in the liver, and unfortunately, they also congest the liver. This liver congestion leads to liver inflammation, which further compromises this already weakened and overburdened organ.

Gallstones clog up the various liver passageways. Some of these stones trickle down through these passageways (called biliary ducts) and find their way into the gall bladder. Once inside the gall bladder, the stones accumulate and grow over time. These stones can become quite large, eventually causing significant health problems. The standard treatment for this problem is the complete removal of the gall bladder—a *cholecystectomy*. This is one of the most common surgeries in the world today, and we are usually told that this will correct the problem. This is a half-truth at best. You need your gall bladder! The gall bladder concentrates the liver's bile by a factor of ten, and in this highly concentrated state, it is capable of properly metabolizing fats, detoxifying the intestines, and carrying out many other important functions. Removing a gall bladder full of gallstones really only attacks the symptoms of the problem because gallstones don't originate in the gall bladder. They originate in the liver.

The liver flush not only empties a gall bladder that may be full of old gallstones, the flush also cleans out biliary passageways full of stones that obstruct, inflame, and hinder the vital functioning of the liver. Clearly, if we can simply get past our aversion to some of the admittedly unpalatable aspects of the liver flush, we may greatly benefit from several of its amazing health-recovering effects.

DETOX STEP #5: The Liver Cleanse

Do this first: Buy 3-4 quarts of unfiltered apple juice (cider) and drink about 14 oz. of it every day for 14 days. Apple juice contains malic acid, which in the body works to soften the gallstones. "Fresh" gallstones are soft, but some people have had old gallstones in their body for years. Over time the stones become hard and potentially sharp-edged. Malic acid changes these hard stones to soft ones, allowing easier passage through the narrow biliary ducts of the body. If you don't have access to good apple juice, simply take malic acid supplements. 1 gram per day of malic acid is an excellent substitute, and should soften the stones just as the apple juice would. Some people actually prefer the malic acid over the apple juice. This includes me. I love drinking apple cider, but drinking cider for two weeks straight is just too much sugar in my diet.

Do this second: On the 15th day, fast completely for the entire day. Drink only water and/or apple juice. At or around 6 pm, mix one tablespoon of magnesium sulfate (Epsom salts) into a cup of apple juice and drink it down. (Using a straw for this not only makes it easier to swallow, it allows for easier ingestion of all of the Epsom salts, which have a very bitter taste.) Magnesium sulfate has some amazing properties, one of which is to dilate vessels in the body. This has a two-fold purpose. One, this dilation has a laxative effect, which should cause you to use the restroom a few times. This is good because your intestines should be clear before the flush occurs anyway. Secondly, magnesium sulfate will also dilate the bile ducts, which will allow the stones—some of which may be quite large—to pass harmlessly through the liver and gall bladder and into the intestines. Take another tablespoon of Epsom salts, mixed with apple juice at around 8 pm. You may have to use the restroom a few more times, but again, you want clean and clear intestines if possible.

Do this third: At 10:00 or 10:30 pm, cut up and juice two lemons (or grapefruit if you prefer) and add this juice to ½ cup of oil— *either olive oil or avocado oil*. Drink it down quickly. Go immediately to bed and lie down on your right side. Try not to move. Go to sleep immediately if you can. In the morning, repeat the Epsom salt and apple juice mixture at 8 am. Repeat again at 10 am. You should be using the restroom throughout the morning and you should see a variety of stones (most of which are green) floating on the surface of the water.

Assess what you have done: Gallstone problems are extremely common. They are a result of a liver overcome with toxins. The word "gallstone" is actually a misnomer in that these are neither stones nor are they formed in the gallbladder. Gallstones are mostly cholesterol, and they form in the liver. The liver

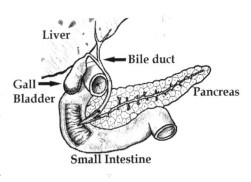

produces about 500 ml of liquid bile every day. When the liver is overburdened with toxins, it produces defective bile which does not remain in liquid form. This defective bile eventually solidifies into what we call *gallstones*. Over time, these stones fill the liver and the various biliary passages. At this point the liver's vital functions are greatly compromised by a now fatty and congested liver, and health problems begin to manifest. These symptoms can be as mild as indigestion or acne. Or they can be as severe as liver cancer and liver failure. Gallstones have also been implicated as a major cause of pancreatic cancer for the same basic reason: a clogged biliary system. Clearly, cleaning out the liver and eliminating this biliary backup is an excellent health-recovering solution.

Why this works: This protocol essentially "tricks" the gallbladder into eliminating its contents. Bile from the liver is stored and concentrated in the gallbladder. When no fats are consumed in the diet, (the fasting on the 15th day) a backpressure is generated in the gallbladder. At this point, it wants to release its pent-up bile. As soon as oil enters the small intestine, the gallbladder will release this bile with considerable force. Since a great deal of oil was consumed, the gallbladder will eject as much of its contents as possible. Since the bile ducts are dilated (due to the Epsom salts) and the gallstones are soft (due to the malic acid), bile and gallstones are ejected out of the gallbladder into the small intestine. The adding of the lemon or grapefruit juice accomplishes two goals. One, either of these juices will help make the swallowing of a ½ cup of oil more palatable. Secondly, by adding a highly acidic substance to the oil, passing through the acidic stomach may occur more quickly, thus reducing or preventing nausea.

Extra: Make sure that after drinking the oil you go immediately to bed on your right side and remain motionless. Try to sleep. The gallbladder evacuates itself only when the body is not moving. If you move a great deal during this time, you will not pass any stones. Also, doing a liver flush releases a considerable amount of toxins into the body at one time. On the day you are actually eliminating your gallstones, you will feel nauseated and lethargic throughout the morning. This is normal. With every visit to the bathroom, you should gradually feel stronger and more energized. Taking several grams of activated charcoal (yes, you read that correctly—grams) during this time can *greatly* reduce the miserable feeling you will have. Also, taking activated charcoal immediately *before* drinking the oil can greatly alleviate the nausea, and this may help you get a better night of sleep. One caution concerning using activated charcoal is that, while it is a powerful toxin neutralizer, it does its job indiscriminately. Activated charcoal will neutralize the effects of most medications, so this must be kept in mind with anyone who is taking daily prescriptions.

Finally, there are a great many liver flush protocols found on the Web. This particular flush is very conservative in comparison to many other flushes in use today. This is by design because a liver cleanse must never be taken lightly. It is highly recommended that you do not try to take short cuts with the apple juice or malic acid. This is particularly true if you have never done a liver cleanse before. Gallstones can be hard, large, and sharp. Only by the use of the apple juice or malic acid can these sharp edges and hardness be reduced to a soft, rubbery stone that is flexible enough to pass through the biliary ducts. These ducts typically have a diameter of only a few (3-7) millimeters. This is about the same diameter as a normal pencil.

REVIEW OF DETOX STEP #5: The Liver Cleanse

Doing a liver cleanse is not like the kidney or thyroid cleanse. It is neither pleasant, nor convenient. However, this cleanse can give amazing results very quickly to the person who does it. Gallstones are a huge health hazard because these stones congest and hinder the function of one of the most important organs in the human body—the liver. Relieving the liver of these stones, which cause blockage, inflammation, and a severe reduction in functionality can bring about enormous health benefits. Bringing relief to your liver can be done very easily, involving only a few key ingredients: apple juice (or malic acid supplements), lemons or grapefruit, oil, Epsom salts, and activated charcoal. While some aspects of this detox protocol are admittedly unpalatable, the end results are well worth any temporary unpleasantness that may be experienced.

TIME/DURATION: After a successful liver flush has been accomplished, gallstones that are too deep in the liver to be removed from this flush will actually move forward and gradually fill the biliary channels and gallbladder again. Doing a monthly liver flush throughout the entire time of your detox is highly recommended in order to keep the healing process moving forward. If you do two consecutive flushes and produce no stones, you have strong evidence that your liver is clean and clear. Doing a maintenance flush once or twice a year following your detox is an excellent solution for retaining a clean liver.

CHAPTER 6

Preparing for a Healing Crisis

I f you have done any research at all into detoxing, you have probably come across terms such as *healing crisis*, *Herxheimer reaction*, or *die off effect*. All of these terms refer to the same thing, which is essentially the body's pushback from detoxing. When a person begins removing old waste products that have been stored deep in tissues, the body will experience negative side effects because the old toxins are again in circulation. If the body is properly prepared for the detox, most of these toxins will be removed from the body. If the body is not properly prepared, such as the kidneys not being cleansed first, many of these toxins in circulation will simply be redistributed and redeposited somewhere else in the body. In either case, the process of detoxing does carry some side effects. These side effects are usually quite temporary, but they can be very unpleasant, so it is a very good idea to be prepared for them in advance.

When I first began to successfully detox, I knew the process was working because I almost always experienced some rather annoying side effects. Many people begin a detox with all sorts of enthusiasm, only to have their enthusiasm extinguished when they experience a healing crisis. Thinking that they have done something wrong, they stop the detoxing process. However, experiencing side effects when you detox is extremely common. It is actually strong evidence that the process is working.

While it is true that detox side effects can range from mild to severe (my side effects usually consisted of nausea, lethargy, swelling, hives, and a very stiff lower back), these side effects can be greatly minimized. Some side effects can even be completely avoided altogether with proper planning and preparation. Here are five practical steps you can take to greatly reduce, or even eliminate altogether, the healing crisis that often accompanies a successful detox.

DETOX STEP #6: Preparing for a Healing Crisis

1. Mind the Order. There is a certain order of steps that a person should take when they detox. I learned this lesson the hard way. I first began my detoxing with the liver flush. The liver flush is an extremely powerful detox protocol, and doing it first was a big mistake. But, I didn't think so at first. I would do a liver flush and feel fantastic... for a few days. *This liver cleanse is incredible. I feel amazing!* Then within a week or so, my lower back would slowly become incredibly stiff and sore. Often times, my abdominal muscles would become very sore as well. This happened so many times that I took this soreness as evidence that my detox was working—and it was. I reasoned that these side effects were just a necessary evil that I had to put up with. This was totally incorrect. Much later on I found out that the kidney cleanse should precede any other detox protocol. Doing a few kidney cleanses before doing any other major detox protocol is a very smart thing to do. This way the kidneys are free and clear of waste, and their functionality is at full strength. A liver flush can cause a great deal of toxins to be liberated inside the body over a very short period of time. This puts a tremendous burden on the kidneys to assist in flushing the toxins out. Only fully functioning kidneys are capable of doing this quickly. My kidneys apparently were not, and the result was soreness and stiffness of the abdominal area and around my lower back. Once I learned that the first cleanse a person should do is the kidney cleanse, this problem went away very quickly. There is a proper order to detoxing, and I believe the kidney cleanse must come first. If you do not obey the order, you might end up paying the consequences. I know I did, and for far too long.

2. Go Low and Slow. As I was experimenting with the thyroid cleanse, I was constantly battling with the side effects of hives and swelling. To make matters worse, this almost always happened at night. So, I would take my supplements, go to bed, and wake up in the morning with a nasty case of hives or swelling. Sometimes the swelling was so bad when I awoke, I was unable to go to work! I looked and felt simply dreadful. This would almost always occur if I took more than the prescribed amount of iodine. I took more iodine than what I was supposed to take because I wanted to speed up the detoxing process. This was another big mistake I frequently made. My body kept telling me to go "low and slow" with the iodine, but I didn't want to listen. However, after a terribly long ground battle with my body, I finally surrendered to it. All of the itchy hives and swelling was just not worth it any longer. Taking supplements in low amounts and slowly building up to higher dosages is the best way to avoid unpleasant side effects. This is especially true with a supplement like iodine and the thyroid cleanse. Iodine is absolutely essential for a good detox, but it is also incredibly powerful and should only be used in *gradually* increasing amounts.

3. Meet the World's Greatest Antidote. As I was making progress in my detoxing, I came across a perplexing paradox. I found that even as I was progressively growing stronger both mentally and physically, my sensitivity to my supplements increased. This was great in one sense because this was evidence that the detox was working. It was also confusing because this required a constant downward adjustment of the dosages of my supplements. This did seem logical. I gradually needed less of my regular supplements to attain the same or increasing level of health and vitality because my system was clearing up. I assumed my absorption of nutrients was increasing, which resulted in my becoming more sensitive to these nutrients. Unfortunately, this also resulted in an unexpected increase in side effects! As I was progressing in my detox, I was more prone to the *healing crisis*, not less. This was indeed a paradox. What was I to do?

I am making such good progress. I can't stop now. But unless I did stop, I would have swelling and hives—almost daily. After a great deal of research, I found an incredibly simple substance—an ancient poison remedy—that was the perfect antidote for my problem. I began taking gradually *increasing* amounts of activated charcoal before I went to bed. Over a matter of just a few days, I found that this simple substance did wonders for preventing the healing crisis side effects of hives and swelling. Activated charcoal is essentially just pure carbon. It can neutralize literally thousands of different types of toxins. This substance can also neutralize many if not most prescription medications, which is one reason why some people are hesitant to use it. I was not taking any medications at the time, so I found this ancient remedy for poisons to be a perfect solution for my perplexing problem. Taking 3 or 4 grams of high quality activated charcoal kept my side effects to a minimum, and this was particularly important when I sometimes pressed all-too-aggressively forward with my detox regimen.

4. Increasing Sensitivity & Dosing Down. I don't know if increasing sensitivity to supplements is everyone's experience when they detox, but as you have already read, it certainly was mine. This was a real challenge at first. I was so used to the normal routine that I had established, I really didn't want to change it. In retrospect, this was the best option however. We are told all the time to "listen to our bodies," and that really is excellent advice, especially when you detox. As you increase in your health and wellness, you will genuinely feel better. This is evidence that your detox is working. This also most likely means that you are more properly absorbing and metabolizing the food and supplements you are taking. So it seems natural that adjustments should be made to your dosage amounts from time to time. This is another good reason to journal your progress. You have a running record of the various amounts of the supplements you are taking. Journaling gives you the ability to know where you are at all times, allowing you to make the proper adjustments whenever needed.

5. A Good Defense is a Good Offense. The last technique I found to be very helpful in reducing the side effects of detoxing is to take a high quality probiotic. I have found the best probiotics to be those that require refrigeration, having at least 100 billion live cultures per capsule. How can a probiotic reduce a healing crisis? Remember that one cause of the negative side effects of a detox is that bad bacteria are being wiped out on a massive scale. These dead bacteria spill their waste products into your system and you experience temporary negative side effects. Unless you repopulate your intestinal tract with the "good guys," the surviving bad bacteria will simply repopulate in your system over time, and you will be back to the same miserable place that you were before. By taking high quality probiotics, you repopulate your system with good bacteria instead, thereby reducing both the frequency and severity of future die off effects.

REVIEW OF DETOX STEP #6: Preparing for a Healing Crisis

Having a mild negative reaction while doing a detox is quite normal. This occurs for many reasons. When a main excretion pathway such as the kidneys are not functioning at full strength, the body is simply not prepared to process the increased levels of toxins that a detox releases. A healing crisis may also occur when the person detoxing is being too aggressive with their supplements, which again results in the body not being adequately prepared to handle the increased volumes of toxins that are now flooding the body's systems. In either of these cases, taking any combination of the precautionary steps discussed in this chapter can vastly reduce the discomfort that a detox often causes. This will result not only in a more pleasant detox experience, it will also encourage you to continue pressing forward until your healing is complete.

TIME/DURATION: A healing crisis can occur at any time during your detox, but usually it occurs at the beginning of the detox. The time and duration required to stave off any healing crisis should be dictated by the frequency and severity of the healing crisis. Usually it will only last for a day or two, but not always. At the height of my problems, I took several grams of activated charcoal on a daily basis for almost a year. Without the charcoal, I would have hives or swelling nearly every day. Reflecting back, I believe that most of these negative reactions that I experienced during my detoxing were due to my own igno-rance, laziness, and lack of patience. As I grew in my understanding of exactly how to detox, these instances occurred with far less frequency. When I really improved in my condition, healing crisis incidents stopped almost completely. Today, of all the five precautionary steps discussed in this chapter, the only one I continue to use on a maintenance basis are the probiotics. These provide a big boost of beneficial intestinal flora, heighten absorption of nutrients, and strengthen my immune system.

CHAPTER 7

The Intestinal Cleanse

O f the four filter cleanses, the intestinal cleanse is perhaps the most difficult to achieve. One reason for this is simply due to the size of the intestines. With the average length of the adult intestine at around 7 meters (23 feet), a great deal of surface area is involved. While cleaning a surface area as large as this is challenging, perhaps the most difficult aspect of clearing the intestines of toxins is the fact that many of these toxins are generated by organisms living inside the intestines. A living, organic adversary is far more formidable than an inorganic one. Toxic metals like mercury and lead are not alive. Yes, these metals settle into tissues and may cause tremendous destruction. However, when you remove the metals, health conditions often improve rapidly. But the intestines often become a home to a great many toxins that are not metals. A person struggling with toxicity very frequently has intestines that have become an ideal habitat for pathogenic bacteria, fungi, and a veritable host of other harmful parasites. These pathogens (or parasites) excrete metabolic waste products that are toxic to humans. Ammonia, alcohol, carbon monoxide, and acetaldehyde are all toxic to humans, and these are the four chemicals that are most commonly excreted into the body by intestinal pathogens. Complicating matters even further, intestinal pathogens specialize in both evading detection and avoiding removal. Even with today's most modern diagnostic tests, the success rate for finding intestinal parasites is a paltry 20-30%.

Not only do pathogenic parasites specialize in evading detection, they are also excellent at adapting to their surroundings. Intestinal parasites have been around for millennia. These pathogens are survivors for several good reasons. They cannot be removed or greatly reduced in numbers permanently by *only* doing intestinal cleanses. The reason for this is because detoxification must occur on a systemic level in order for permanent changes to happen. Detoxing only the intestines and ignoring the kidneys, thyroid, and liver may bring temporary relief. But without a systemic change, the intestines will eventually revert back to their old toxic state. Parasites are fighters. When they find themselves in a hostile environment, they retreat into their hiding places (the mucus layer of the intestines) or assume some inactive form, such as a *spore*. After the intestinal cleanse is completed, their hostile environment has been removed, and the parasites emerge from their hiding places, and inactive forms, to continue their destructive work.

To illustrate the point, let's review just the essential phases of general toxicity. We'll examine mercury metal in this example because it is such a pervasive problem world-wide. Please don't take this personally, but we'll use *you* as the person of interest in this story.

You were born with mercury problems because your mother and grandmother had "silver amalgam" fillings in their mouths. This mercury was passed to you through fetal blood and breast milk. Your thyroid was the first filter to be affected by this mercury, as this damage actually began before you were born. As you grew up, you had minor thyroid problems, though you didn't know about it at the time. You did struggle with acne, fatigue, and weight-related issues, but you assumed that this was due to your genetics and food choices. *You simply are a teenager with a slow metabolism, and this has nothing to do with a thyroid problem—right?*

Years pass, and the weakened thyroid's relationship with the liver begins to show. The liver requires a generous supply of the thyroid hormone thyroxine in order to properly process cholesterol, and to produce bile. Without an adequate supply of thyroxine, cholesterol levels in the liver rise. This causes blood cholesterol levels to become elevated. The thyroxine hormone shortage also causes the liver to produce defective bile, which results in gallstones. These gallstones begin to cause small amounts of blockage in the liver, slowly compromising its functioning. The gallstones also affect pancreatic function because some stones inadvertently tumbled too close to the pancreatic duct and slightly blocked this juncture. Notice the main bile duct and pancreatic duct are joined together as they connect to the small intestine. (Gallstones have been implicated as one cause of pancreatic cancer, and this design feature is probably one reason why.)

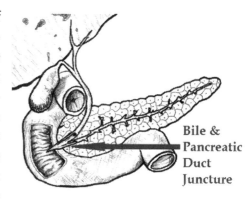

Bile & Pancreatic Duct Juncture

Normally, your liver should produce about 500 ml of free-flowing bile per day. But the gallstones have reduced this volume to an unknown amount. Some of these stones also found their way into your gall bladder, where a sort of "snowball" effect occurred, and the stones grew larger. Over time, these stones grew so large that they could not be released by the gall bladder any longer. They were simply too big for the bile duct. As a result of all of this, you are now experiencing abdominal pain, stiffness around the joints and shoulders, digestive disturbances, skin eruptions, blood-sugar issues, and cholesterol problems. Unfortunately, your problems are just getting started.

Downstream from all of this trouble, more health issues are beginning to develop. Because of the bile drought, the intestinal pH (the acid-alkaline balance) has been significantly altered. This happened because the bile, which is strongly alkaline, was no longer flowing in the amounts needed. Without this constant coating of alkaline bile, the intestines switched from their normally alkaline state to an acidic state. This switch caused the good intestinal bacteria to die in large numbers, but allowed the harmful bacteria to flourish. Intestinal fungal overgrowth also occurred because of this altered pH. Intestinal pathogen populations grew to such an extent that the main toxins released by these pathogens—ammonia, alcohol, carbon monoxide, and acetaldehyde—are now posing several serious health threats. The liver, already overtaxed with toxins and burdened with gallstones, cannot begin to process and neutralize these new toxins effectively. In a desperate attempt to protect itself from these parasitically-produced toxins, the intestinal tract vastly increases its own production of mucus. This mucus does offer some protection from the toxins, but it also serves as an excellent hiding place for the parasites when you try to cleanse your intestines. The mucus buildup also prevents the proper absorption of nutrients into the body, and so even as you are gaining more and more weight, areas of your body are actually starved for nutrients. This results in a further weakening of your body, which is already rapidly deteriorating in health.

Yes, this is a rather bleak picture, but I believe it is an entirely accurate one. I should know. This is what happened to me. My problems began with mercury before I was born, and this poisoning triggered a series of harmful conditions and events that ultimately caused the collapse of my health. I believe this same health collapse is currently happening to countless people around the world right now. Although this situation is dire, it is not irrevocable. Detoxing through a series of logical steps can reverse much, if not all of this damage. I did it, and so can you.

True systemic change begins when the kidney filters are cleared so that waste is eliminated quickly and efficiently. The next step is to clean the thyroid so that proper metabolic functions are restored and so that the liver is properly supported by vital thyroid hormones. This can be done while concurrently cleaning the liver so that whole-body detoxification proceeds in an efficient manner. A clean liver will produce ample volumes of alkaline bile, which assist in cholesterol metabolism, the stabilizing of intestinal pH, and the cleaning of the intestinal walls. Clean intestinal walls allow for better absorption of food nutrients. When food nutrient absorption is high, a person's health and energy levels soar, and there is very little food left behind to feed intestinal pathogens.

DETOX STEP #7: The Intestinal Cleanse

Do this first: Buy a container of high quality food-grade Diatomaceous Earth (DE), an anti-fungal supplement, and a high quality probiotic. Begin taking your DE by mixing one heaping teaspoon of this chalky powder with juice or in a smoothie. DE really has no flavor, and simply mixing it with water results in a drink that has a chalky texture. This may irritate your throat. I prefer my DE drink at night, though some people state that this has a tendency to keep them awake. Whether it is night or morning, you should drink your DE juice or smoothie every day. Over the course of a few weeks, try to work up to one or two heaping *tablespoons* of DE every day in your juice or smoothie. Expect to see and smell some rather pungent solid waste being removed from your body, especially during these first initial months of the protocol. This is completely natural, as your body is eliminating a great deal of old, encrusted waste from the intestinal walls.

Do this second: After a week or so of taking the DE, begin taking your anti-fungal supplement in addition to your DE drink. Begin with just one pill of the supplement and slowly work up to the maximum dosage level as shown on the label. If you find that you cannot tolerate the maximum level, find an upper level of dosage that you can tolerate and stay at this level until your intestinal cleanse is completed.

Do this third: After two weeks on your intestinal cleanse, you can begin taking your probiotic. Again, start with just one pill of the supplement and slowly work up to the maximum dosage level as shown on the label. Again, if you find that you cannot tolerate the maximum level, find an upper level of dosage that you can tolerate.

Optional: As an additional support to your intestinal cleanse, you may try taking some essential oils. Oregano, peppermint, clove, and cinnamon oil all have powerful anti-fungal, antiviral, and antibiotic qualities. Oregano is by far the most powerful of all the essential oils in the anti-fungal category, but it is also the most difficult one to take in pure form. It is highly irritating on the skin and should always be mixed with another oil. Peppermint, clove, and cinnamon oils are less harsh, and can be taken directly with water. Essential oils are extremely powerful and not everyone tolerates these oils equally well. I have found each of these oils to be tremendously helpful with reestablishing normal intestinal functioning, but a certain amount of testing and experimentation with essential oils is required. Start with just one of the three oils and mix 3-7 drops in equal amounts with an inert oil (olive, avocado, or coconut oil) in a 00 or 000-sized vegetable capsule. Swallow immediately as the oils typically will dissolve the capsule in as little time as a minute.

Assess what you have done: As has already been mentioned, the intestinal cleanse is the most difficult one to achieve because a large variety of variables are in play. A toxic intestinal tract is a multi-level problem. But you have taken a multi-level approach to attacking this problem of encrusted waste on the intestinal walls, poor levels of healthy bacteria in the intestines, and high levels of pathogenic bacteria and fungi. Each of these protocols address a specific issue, but this cleanse does require constant monitoring and frequent adjustments to dosages. Even so, I have found the intestinal cleanse to provide rapid and powerful health benefits, some of which may be experienced in as little time as one week.

Why This Works: The Diatomaceous Earth (DE) accomplishes two very important objectives of the intestinal cleanse. It cleans the intestinal walls of excess mucus (a habitat for many pathogens), and it is able to kill many of the pathogenic organisms living in the intestines. It is able to do this because DE has a negative charge (chemically speaking) and pathogens have a positive charge. Therefore, the DE attaches to the pathogens, but leaves the good intestinal bacteria unharmed. DE is an exceptionally fine powder, and it is exceedingly hard. This makes DE a powerful abrasive, and its negative charge causes it to be attracted to the pathogens, which it literally shreds to pieces on contact. Microscopic parasites have no defense against it, and this is why DE actually has a rather long history of being used as an intestinal cleanse for both humans and livestock. It is very efficient while at the same time being extremely cost-effective.

As the DE gently but efficiently removes parasites and excess mucus from intestinal walls, the now freely-flowing bile—due to your liver flushes—assists in the removal of parasites and heavy metals. The body's most powerful antioxidant and natural chelator is *glutathione*. This chemical flows with the bile, attracting and neutralizing toxins all along its path. The bile is also strongly alkaline, another important feature which helps to shift the intestinal environment from a sickly acidic state (which is friendly to pathogens) to a healthy alkaline state (which is hostile to pathogens). Further aiding in the healing and cleaning process of the intestines is the anti-fungal and probiotic supplements that are being taken. Probiotics are essential for an intestinal cleanse because they bring multitudes of good bacteria to the intestines, where they should thrive in this newly cleaned and properly pH-balanced environment.

REVIEW OF DETOX STEP #7: The Intestinal Cleanse

The fourth and final filter that needs cleaning during a detox are the intestines. The intestinal cleanse is probably the most difficult one to achieve because of the overall area that needs to be cleaned, and because the intestines are home to living organisms that produce toxins. Cleaning the intestines first begins with food grade Diatomaceous Earth. This exceedingly fine and hard substance has been used as an anti-parasite food additive for both humans and livestock for generations. It literally scrapes the intestines clean of harmful parasites and excess mucus in a safe and gentle manner. Since the liver has already been cleaned of excess gallstones, normal bile flow has been reestablished. Bile is strongly alkaline, and the newly flowing bile will help the intestines to slowly shift from their sickly acidic state to the normal, healthful alkaline state. Bile can also kill pathogenic microorganisms, which further cleans the intestines. Finally, by taking a high quality probiotic, you are making great strides towards ensuring that the intestines are repopulated with non-pathogenic, healthy flora which assists the human body with several important functions, including aiding in digestion, boosting the immune system, and assisting in the production of vitamins.

TIME/DURATION: The intestinal cleanse can begin concurrently with the thyroid and liver cleanse, though this may be difficult for some individuals due to the sheer volume of toxins that are being eliminated. I recommend doing an intestinal cleanse for a minimum of 3-6 months.

CHAPTER 8

Chelation

C helation is the practice of using supplements to assist the body in removing heavy metals such as mercury and lead. This assistance is necessary because if the body cannot excrete a toxic metal upon exposure,
it does the next best thing, which is to store the toxin deep within tissues
where it can do as little damage as possible. This does not work extremely well
with mercury and lead, which is one reason why these metals are notorious for
causing mental disorders. If a toxin can get into the brain and do damage, it
certainly can get into any other area of the body and do damage there as well.
Powerful toxins like mercury and lead simply overwhelm the body's natural
defenses. This is why the body needs help in eliminating certain toxins, and
chelation is able to provide this help.

The body produces a variety of "natural chelators," but its most powerful
chelation substance is a molecule called *glutathione*. This molecule is produced
by every cell in the body. Not surprisingly, most of the body's glutathione is
produced in the liver. Glutathione has several important roles. It renders free
radicals harmless, it boosts the immune system, and glutathione can even bind
to a toxin like mercury and escort it out of the body. But simply taking chelation
supplements, including synthetic glutathione, is not usually the answer for any
adult who wants to detox. If that were the case, than detoxing would simply be
a matter of taking chelating supplements every day until your system clears out.
I know all too well the futility of this, because I tried to do it myself for years.

POTENTIALLY TOXIC ELEMENTS (3-Year-Old ♀)				
	RESULT µg/g	RANGE	PERCENTILE	
			68th	95th
Aluminum	38.0	<12.0		
Antimony	0.17	<0.080		
Arsenic	0.043	<0.120		
Bismuth	0.84	<2.0		
Cadmium	0.21	<0.150		
Lead	1.3	<2.0		
Mercury	0.14	<1.10		
Uranium	0.098	<0.060		
Nickel	1.100	<0.40		
Silver	17	<0.10		
Tin	0.61	<0.30		
Titanium	5.0	<1.00		
Total Toxic Representation				

When I first discovered that mercury metal is transmitted generationally from mothers with mercury to their children, I sent out hair samples from both of my children to a lab for analysis. I knew for a fact that my children's mother and maternal grandmother had mercury amalgam fillings. I did not know about their maternal great-grandmother because she wore dentures for a good portion of her life. But seeing that both the mother and grandmother had mercury fillings (and both had some rather serious health issues of their own), I knew that my kids were at least 3rd generation mercury toxic. The lab results of their hair analysis confirmed this. Shown here is the data from my three-year-old daughter's first hair sample. These numbers were horrible, and I immediately began giving both of my children very conservative dosage levels of chelation supplements. Mixing these supplements with either milk or juice, I gave this "vitamin drink" (as I called it) to both of my children. I did this for 16 months and then sent in another hair sample for analysis. The data from this second hair analysis was very encouraging. There was a 36% drop in overall toxicity. I took this as powerful evidence that the chelation was working, and continued on this simple supplement protocol.

Toxin	Original Level	After 16 Months	% Increase or Decrease
Aluminum	38.0	25.0	34% Decrease
Antimony	0.17	0.027	84% Decrease
Arsenic	0.043	0.049	14% Increase
Bismuth	0.84	0.091	89% Decrease
Cadmium	0.21	0.061	71% Decrease
Lead	1.30	0.85	35% Decrease
Mercury	0.14	0.27	92% Increase
Uranium	0.098	0.16	63% Increase
Nickel	1.10	0.36	67% Decrease
Silver	17.0	0.14	99% Decrease
Tin	0.61	0.25	59% Decrease
Titanium	5.0	2.10	58% Decrease

Toxin	Original Level	After 46 Months	% Increase or Decrease
Aluminum	38.0	11.0	71% Decrease
Antimony	0.17	<0.01	99% Decrease
Arsenic	0.043	0.045	5% Increase
Bismuth	0.84	0.013	98% Decrease
Cadmium	0.21	0.016	92% Decrease
Lead	1.30	0.10	92% Decrease
Mercury	0.14	<0.003	99% Decrease
Uranium	0.098	0.14	43% Increase
Nickel	1.10	0.18	84% Decrease
Silver	17.0	0.02	99% Decrease
Tin	0.61	0.03	95% Decrease
Titanium	5.0	0.31	94% Decrease

After thirty more months of having my kids take their daily "vitamin drink," I sent two more hair samples to the lab for analysis. When I got the results back a few weeks later, I was blown away. After four years of mild chelation, both of my kids showed tremendous improvement. Here is the data from my daughter's second hair analysis. There was a whopping 73% reduction in overall toxicity. My daughter was now a happy and very healthy seven-year-old girl. The only thing infectious about her was her smile. *The chelation had worked.*

Curiously, while both children received tremendous benefits from this very simple chelation protocol, I did not. I took the same supplements that they did during this time period, but my health continued to plummet. After a significant amount of research, I came to a very simple conclusion as to why the chelation did not work for me.

My children got a tremendous benefit from the chelating supplements because they were young, and their kidneys, thyroid, liver, and intestines were not nearly as toxic as mine. However, in a very real sense, my body was too polluted to receive the benefits of the chelating supplements. I didn't think that my liver was "too far gone" to get any benefit from chelating, but after four long years of trying, it was obvious I was doing something terribly wrong. Once I learned the simple truth that the liver filter needed to be cleaned first *before* chelating, and implemented this truth, I began to rapidly recover my health.

DETOX STEP #8: Chelation

Do this first: Purchase a chelating supplement. There are several excellent chelating supplements available, and each has their advantages and disadvantages. After a considerable amount of research, I chose to use Chelorex and Detox Max Plus (see Appendix). I saw excellent results from both of these products. Whatever chelating substance you choose, I recommend starting with a very low dosage of the supplement and slowly working up to the maximum dosage level as shown on the label. If you find that you cannot tolerate the maximum level, find an upper level dosage that you can tolerate and stick with it for the duration of the time you choose to chelate.

Why This Works: A body that is extremely toxic needs outside help, and chelating substances can provide this help. Working within a body that has its four filters cleaned, or at least are in the process of being cleaned, chelating substances can work in conjunction with the body's systems to speed up the cleaning—and therefore the healing—process.

REVIEW OF DETOX STEP #8: Chelation

Some people look at the term "chelation" with a certain degree of fear and trepidation, as if it were some strange new health practice. This fear is completely unfounded. Chelation can be done with very simple supplements and foods. Moreover, the human body produces the most powerful chelating substance available—for free. The problem is that this substance, glutathione, is produced in massive amounts by the liver, and it travels in the bile. If the liver is toxic and full of gallstones, the glutathione can't get to its intended destinations in the volumes that a toxic body requires. For young children, doing a kidney, thyroid, and intestinal cleanse may be possible, depending upon their ages. But a liver cleanse would be very difficult for a young child. However, using chelation supplements is an excellent alternative for young children. For adults however, these four cleanses are all essential if you truly want to get the maximum benefit from the chelating substances you are taking. Clean the filters first, and then put in the supplements. This is not to say that putting high quality supplements into a body that has toxicity issues is a complete waste of money, but it is often an extremely inefficient use of both supplements and money.

TIME/DURATION: There are a large variety of chelating substances available on the market, and each one has certain dosages and time frames that they operate within. I suggest keeping to the parameters set by the particular product, and repeat as needed. I personally chelated for several years, but as I have already indicated, I did it in the wrong way. After cleaning out my own filters, particularly my liver, I found chelation brought very significant health improvements within just a few months.

CHAPTER 9

Dietary Changes and Challenges

I f you have read many books or articles on detoxing, you may already have some preconceived notions concerning what this chapter will discuss. Whenever people consider doing a detox, they usually come face to face with certain eating habits that—putting it mildly—may require some adjustment. This chapter is no exception to this, but the dietary changes I discuss here may surprise you.

Dietary changes are usually required for a good detox because most of us eat too much sugar and too many processed foods. Large quantities of sugar and processed foods require a significant amount of additional work from an already overtaxed digestive system. But dietary changes do not mean that you have to implement new eating habits that only a goat would enjoy. If you are like me, you have seen detox diets by the dozens and many of these sound, look, and probably taste the same. "*Eat only whole foods. Stay away from red meat. Avoid white flour. All vegetables taste awesome if you prepare them the right way. Forget every type of sweet you ever enjoyed from here on out. Don't even think about coffee, even black coffee. Avoid any tea except the herbal teas. Never mind the fact that many herbal teas taste like diluted perfume...you just have to remember how good these teas are for you.*"

Most of us have heard these sorts of things before. This is not to say that many detox diets are unhealthy. Many if not most of these diets probably are very healthy. How could your body not improve in its condition if you tripled the amount of vegetables that you eat on a daily basis? I tried some of these diets, and I admit I did get a health boost from them. My problem is I couldn't stick with the diet. I just didn't like to eat this way for too long. The food simply did not taste that great to me. And after a short while, I was back to my old diet again. I love bacon and eggs for breakfast, and I deliberately put way too much butter on my toast. This is the way I like to eat.

Well, eventually I found out that most of the foods that I was eating I could keep right on eating. I didn't want to give up on those foods, and I found I didn't have to. However, I need to quickly add that I did make some dietary changes as I was detoxing. But these changes—all of which were good—were made mostly because I wanted to make these changes myself, and not because I was told I needed to make the changes. Allow me to explain what I mean by this.

After I finally learned how to detox the right way, many changes began to occur in my system. Several of these changes were completely unexpected. One significant change was with food. My desire for certain foods changed dramatically. I found that I enjoyed the taste of whole foods much more than I ever had before. Meanwhile, highly processed foods that typically came out of a box often tasted either very bland, or had an annoying chemical taste to it. Processed foods that I used to enjoy simply did not taste that great anymore. Neither were these foods satisfying. This was also true concerning restaurant food. I still loved a good cheeseburger and fries, but usually only when I cooked these myself, using real cheese, healthy oils, and high grade beef. Most restaurant food tasted like a cheap substitute to real food, which I suppose in many ways it was. In contrast to this, homemade food usually tasted amazing! This was now the food I craved. So, over a relatively short period of time, I began to make some fairly significant changes in my diet that were very positive. These changes came from a change in desire, and that made all the difference to me. There were only a few foods (mostly highly processed foods) that I gave up on with any real regret. Many of these foods contained either high fructose corn syrup (HFCS) or monosodium glutamate (MSG).

As has already been mentioned, HFCS was found to contain trace amounts of mercury back in 2009. Mercury was an element that I had specifically targeted for excretion during my detox. I wanted absolutely no part of mercury metal in my system any longer. Unfortunately, the artificial sweetener HFCS is found in an enormous number of foods, some of which were personal favorites of mine. But since a "safe" amount of mercury does not exist, I walked away from HFCS permanently, along with all of the foods in which it was found.

Other foods that I somewhat regretfully walked away from were various favorites that contained a significant amount of monosodium glutamate (MSG). This chemical food additive is a popular flavor enhancer with no less than fifteen aliases! Obviously, certain food manufacturers want to enjoy the benefits of using MSG in their foods without the consumers being aware of this use. I had found over the years that I was chemically sensitive to MSG, but I oftentimes ignored the symptoms of hives and occasional swelling. This was now going to stop. So I also abandoned MSG foods and my body certainly benefited from this abdication. These two food groups I gave up because I basically had to. Most other foods I gave up by choice, and some of these foods surprised me.

I have always had a sweet tooth, and I have always enjoyed eating large amounts of bread. I have loved these types of foods for as long as I can remember. After I began making significant progress with cleaning out all four of my filters, I found that my desire for breads and sweets was *significantly* diminished. For example, there was a time in my life when I could drink a half liter of soda without even thinking about it. Who doesn't like soda, especially with a slice of pizza or with buttery popcorn? A long while ago, I used to drink soda like it was water. However, after a year or so of effective detoxing, drinking soda became less and less attractive to me. It didn't matter what I was eating for the meal, drinking a soda along with the meal just did not sound appealing. Soda tasted far too sweet for my tastes now. On the rare occasion that I did drink soda, I found that only a very small amount was satisfying. What had changed? It wasn't the soda that had changed, it was me.

There are some very good biochemical reasons for these changes. I believe cleaning out the liver and bile ducts were contributing factors in this because the bile duct joins the pancreatic duct just before it interfaces with the small intestine. This clearing away of blockage allowed for pancreatic juices to more easily reach their required destinations. Perhaps even more importantly, the thyroid hormone thyroxin directly influences pancreatic function. Clean out the liver and thyroid, and the pancreas improves in its functioning. In over-simplified terms, I was able to process sugars far more efficiently with the liver and thyroid filters clear, and so a little soda went a long way now. Furthermore, with the intestines getting cleaned up nicely as they were being detoxed, parasitic organisms living in the intestines—all of which love to eat sugar and were doubtless a driving force behind the breads and sweets cravings—were dying off in large numbers. With less parasitic mouths to feed, my desire for breads and sweets was also greatly diminished.

REVIEW OF DETOX STEP #9: Dietary Changes and Challenges

Doing an effective detox does require some dietary changes to be made. Even before a person detoxes, they should listen carefully to how their body reacts to certain foods. Any foods that elicit an allergic response or cause digestive disturbances should be avoided, at least temporarily, until the detox is completed. In addition to these deliberate changes, other positive dietary changes may occur spontaneously as the food desires of the person doing the detox also change. These changes in desire are normal. As the four filters of the body increasingly become clear of obstructions and contaminants, the body is able to process food much more efficiently. The detox appears to affect how the body communicates internally. This improved communication results in over-all positive changes in food desires. These changes should be expected during and immediately following a good detox.

TIME/DURATION: Changes in food desires are natural during a good detox, and are a strong indicator that the detox is effectively making positive changes in the various systems of the body. A general shift from processed foods to whole foods, and from high doses of sugar to lower amounts of sugar are excellent changes that should be pursued ongoing without any limit to time or duration.

CHAPTER 10

Exercise and Rest

This tenth step in the *12 Step Detox* is one that we all know we need to take, but it is something that often gets placed at the end of our priorities. This was certainly true for me. Before I got sick, I loved being active. Working out in the gym, running, playing basketball, swimming, and biking were all important parts of my physical conditioning. However, when my health started to collapse, I was far less motivated in this area of my life. I just didn't feel like being active the way I used to be anymore. The precious little energy that I did have was devoted to my family and career. My body certainly did not benefit from this lack of exercising, but there was little I could do about it. I used to have a strong desire to exercise, but this desire was slowly diminishing right along with my health. I simply did not have the energy to exercise, and if you don't have the energy, you don't exercise.

I knew I was in bad shape, but I didn't really grasp how far I had fallen until I had my testosterone level checked. I had been seeing a sports doctor for some time because of a chronically sore back. I casually mentioned to him that in addition to my back problems, my overall energy level was very low. I was always tired, and rarely seemed to have any spare energy. I thought perhaps this was just old age creeping up on me, prematurely. The doctor suggested that I get my total testosterone level (T-level) checked, which I promptly did. Weeks later, when I presented the doctor with this lab information, the conversation went something like this:

"Well Chris...your T-level is at a 182. For a person of your age and build, I would say that a level of 300 is your bare minimum. We have got to find a way to increase this. Should this level fall to, say 160, you could be in a life-threatening situation."

That statement got my attention. *Life-threatening? That did not sound good.* Not too long after this rather depressing conversation, I began to see some success with my detoxing. Fast forward about a year and a half and I was back in the doctor's office with a new testosterone report. I was feeling much better due to the detox and I wanted to show the doctor my results. My T-level was now at a semi-respectable 283, a 55% increase from my previous level. I continued to detox, and continued to improve both physically and mentally. Six months later I again had my T level checked. It was now at 306. By the time I had finished detoxing, my T-level stood at a whopping 512. My testosterone had increased 181% without using any synthetics or artificial supplements. *Absolutely amazing.*

What was the reason for this dramatic change? This is a very good question and one that I spent a significant amount of time investigating in the research. The best answer I could come up with was that toxicity had caused my body to be in a constant state of inflammation. Toxins irritate tissues, which become inflamed. This inflammation was everywhere—muscles, joints, tendons, organs—because the toxins were everywhere!

One of the main hormones the body produces to combat inflammation is *cortisol*. This very powerful hormone is quite effective at reducing inflammation. However, and this is the key point, the body produces cortisol in inverse proportions to testosterone. High cortisol production means low testosterone production. This made sense to me. After all, high testosterone levels would give a body that was already experiencing high levels of inflammation an even greater opportunity to become inflamed. Because I was now effectively detoxing, this whole situation was reversed. Detoxing significantly reduced my overall internal inflammation, which reduced my body's need for cortisol. This reduction in cortisol allowed my body to produce greatly needed testosterone, causing my T-levels to soar.

As was noted in the previous chapter, one of the wonderful aspects I experienced in doing a detox is that my food desires began to change. I believe a good detox should change your desires, because as your body changes for the better, so does your mind. Well, the same is true for my desire and ability to exercise. As my internal system slowly got cleared up, my desire and ability to exercise reawakened. Actually, this is a bit of an understatement. When you move from a T-level of 182 to 512, you *need* to exercise. Getting a good workout was not only my joy again, it was an absolute necessity. I was at a point now where I actually needed a rigorous workout a few times a week in order to feel good. This is not to say that I suddenly began living in a gym. I did not. I found that only a few hours a week were necessary for me to bring my fitness and conditioning to a satisfactory level. As strange as this sounds, my exercising actually helped me rest and enjoy levels of relaxation that I had not experienced in years. I slept more soundly now, and yet required less sleep.

REVIEW OF DETOX STEP #10: Exercise and Rest

Doing an effective detox will boost your energy. A portion of this energy should be devoted to building up your body again. For some people, this is a very easy thing to do. For others, the act of exercising in a vigorous, methodical manner is a matter of pure willpower. If you feel you fit in this second group, don't follow your heart in this matter. *Lead your heart.* As you detox, you should gradually begin to feel less tired. Use some of this newly available energy to exercise in ways that you enjoy. This can have a compounding effect where success leads to more success. Detoxing improves how you feel by giving you more energy, which can be used for regular exercise. This exercise will improve both how you look and how you feel on a daily basis.

TIME/DURATION: Getting an appropriate amount of exercise every week is an excellent practice that works very well alongside your detox regimen. As such, there should be no limit to the time or duration of this, as exercising should be a regular part of everyone's life.

CHAPTER 11

Pacing

Pacing your detox requires planning, patience, and a great deal of careful listening. When I say "listening" I am referring to listening to your body. How is your body responding to the detox protocols you are implementing? It's a good idea to keep in mind the notion that even if you are doing everything right, you most likely will experience some form of healing crisis. While everyone who detoxes has one main goal in common (get the poisons out), each person also has different specific needs. Individuals often demonstrate slightly different responses to detox protocols. This is why creating a single detox schedule and then putting it into action with the expectation that it will be universally compatible with everyone is not realistic. However, there are certain trends in detoxing that should be recognized, and minding the order of detox protocols is one such trend that should at least be acknowledged, if not directly followed.

As has already been mentioned, when I first began to detox, I did many things wrong. I began with taking a toxin inventory through a hair analysis (right), and then I plunged right into taking chelation supplements (wrong). After a great deal of time and money spent with seeing no progress, I tried doing monthly liver cleanses (right), but I did these cleanses for over a year without ever doing a kidney cleanse (wrong). I did *not* mind the order of detoxing because I did not know that an order even existed! Now I know better, and you the reader are the beneficiary of this knowledge.

But how exactly would I schedule my detox, and what kind of overlap and pacing should I have with the various protocols? This is a very good question. The answer is it depends upon the unique needs of the individual. Some people are extremely toxic and desperately need to utilize all twelve steps. But, because of their extreme toxicity, these people need to take extra care. Too much overlap of the steps may put too much of a strain on their system, thereby incurring the body's wrath with many and varied healing crisis episodes. This certainly was my experience. I needlessly suffered from a variety of healing crisis episodes until I learned how to correctly "mind the order" of detox protocols. I also started actually listening to my body. Knowing the correct order of detoxing and listening to my body allowed me to pace my detox in a manner that was right for me. Though I made many mistakes along the way, I finally figured out how to correctly detox. If I could start all over again from the very beginning, my pacing schedule would look something like this:

	Jan	Feb	Mar	Apr	May	Jun	Jul	Aug	Sep	Oct	Nov	Dec	Jan	Feb	Mar
Kidney Cleanse	X	X	X	X			X				X				X
Thyroid Cleanse		X	X	X	X	X	X	X	X	X	X	X	X	X	X
Liver Cleanse			X	X		X		X		X		X		X	
Intestinal Cleanse				X	X	X	X	X	X	X	X				
Chelation Supplements					X	X	X	X	X	X	X	X			
Toxin Inventory	X						X						X		

As previously mentioned, the toxin inventory should be the official start of anyone's detox. This inventory provides the baseline data that will be of utmost value as the detox moves forward and a person begins to recover their health. The first kidney cleanse should occur immediately after this, and this cleanse should be repeated for several months to insure this vital elimination pathway is clear. The thyroid cleanse can begin around the second month, and the first liver flush at the third month. After progress has been made in these areas, the intestinal cleanse may commence, with chelating supplements taken a month or so after that. I like the staggered start of this sample detox schedule because it gives the body time and resources to properly manage the huge increase of toxins that are being liberated from the body's tissues.

I recommend taking a second toxin inventory about six months after the detox has officially begun. Anytime sooner may not show any significant improvement, particularly if you are using the hair analysis as a diagnostic tool. But waiting an entire year before taking a second toxin inventory may cause you to miss valuable data that should have been collected earlier.

This 15-month detox schedule contains all of the elements needed for a comprehensive whole-body detox, with careful attention given towards cleaning the four main filtration areas, and supporting the protocol cleanses with both adequate supplements and time.

REVIEW OF DETOX STEP #11: Pacing

Putting together a schedule that paces a person's detox is best done by the individual who is detoxing. They know what their body is telling them and what protocols and dosage levels of supplements they are able to tolerate. After years of research and personal experimentation, I feel the pacing schedule shown in this chapter may be a good place to start for many people because this schedule minds the correct order of detox protocols and introduces new protocols gradually, on a staggered basis. However, the final authority of the pacing should rest with the individual who is detoxing, because they know their own bodies and are best able to determine what adjustments need to be made as they move forward in their detox.

TIME/DURATION: The time needed to complete a detox is entirely up to the individual. Some people have an enormous need to detox and therefore the time needed will be significantly greater than for an individual with only minor detox issues. If a person wishes to complete all 12 steps of this detox, I believe

12 to 15 months is an adequate period of time to accomplish this. If the person still feels they have lingering issues after their first detox, this individual should commence a second detox that has been modified to address the specific issues that continue to demand attention.

CHAPTER 12

Reflection

The final stage in the *12 Step Detox* is one of reflection and review. This last stage requires a careful analysis of the data collected (from hair analysis forms and from personal journal entries) and a thoughtful introspection on how one is currently feeling. If you completed a 15-month detox similar to the schedule shown in the previous chapter, you may feel vastly different from how you felt before you began your detox. *How do I feel now compared to how I felt before I began my detox? In what areas have I improved? What areas, if any, still require some attention? Does the data from my hair analyses and journal entries correlate with how I am currently feeling?* These are all excellent questions a person who has completed a detox should ask themselves. Reviewing and reflecting on this information can give you strong direction with where you should go next.

The reflection step may indeed be the final step of your detox, but not necessarily. I found that once I finished my detox, there were still some lingering issues that required attention. I suppose this is completely normal, though I am not entirely certain why. One possible scenario that must be considered is the issue of permanent damage. *Did my prolonged exposure to toxins over the years cause permanent damage within my liver, kidneys, thyroid, or in some other vital area?* While this is a definite possibility with everyone, our response to the issues will probably be the same. If we have lingering issues, we should focus on those protocols that address those issues.

Another possible reason for a continued need to detox is that the first round of detoxing simply wasn't complete. Either there are some heavy metals still deeply buried in tissues that require removal, or there are biologically-produced toxins coming from Candida or some other parasite that still needs attention. In either case, the answer is the same. Focus on repeating those protocols that are appropriate for addressing the remaining problem. For example, even though my "official" detoxing ended years ago, I still find that doing an occasional kidney flush (by occasional I mean 3 or 4 per year) to be very helpful with lower back stiffness. I also do a liver cleanse once or twice a year for general maintenance. For me, this is just a good precautionary measure, but for others, it may be a necessity. For example, I have a friend who does a liver cleanse anytime his cholesterol levels creep close to the 200 level. He says that the flushes bring an immediate impact on these levels, reducing his cholesterol count by 20-30 points.

REVIEW OF DETOX STEP #12: Reflection

Reviewing and reflecting on both the data collected and how your physical and mental states have improved by detoxing is extremely valuable. I have found that as I detoxed, I would periodically review the data from my journal entries and from my hair analysis forms to gain perspective, and to get a clearer picture of where I thought I was heading. This reviewing and reflecting on the data also greatly encouraged me. I needed this encouragement. Some aspects of detoxing are extremely private. I usually didn't tell anyone that I was in the middle of a kidney cleanse, nor was I in the habit of showing friends the results of a successful liver flush. That kind of information is not what most people would consider "socially acceptable." But as I improved in my health, it became increasingly evident that something very good was happening to me. My appearance was different, and my actions were different. These changes were very encouraging, and really spurred me on to continue my detox until I reached a level of wellness that was truly satisfying. Detoxing is work. It takes a committed effort. While its rewards are almost too numerous to mention, detoxing does take you through some dark valleys at times. Far too many people give up on their detox and stay in that dark valley. My encouragement to anyone doing a detox is to keep climbing the mountain until you reach the top. You can do it! And when you reach the top, you will see that the view from the summit is simply spectacular.

Appendix

Chapter 1: A History of Toxicity

Mercury toxicity is a far bigger problem than what most people realize. Mercury's unique ability to cross critical blood barriers allows this poison to be transmitted through the generations. This horrible ability is unprecedented. Many years ago I compiled a lengthy list of many of the wretched health problems that scholarly research directly or indirectly linked to mercury toxicity. This list is shown here.

Neurological & Cardiovascular

Depression, detached from reality, brain fog, memory lapses, tremors, epilepsy, numb extremities, cramps, twitches, jitteriness, restless leg syndrome, fragile nerves, loss of sensory sensitivity, unexplained chest pain, unexplained tachycardia.

Collagen

Arthritis, frequent or constant pain, discomfort in joints; upper and/or lower back pain.

Immunological

Weakened immune system, ears, nose, and throat issues; autoimmune disorders, including MS, ALS, and lupus; Diabetes, psoriasis, certain types of arthritis, Epstein-Barr, cancer, AIDS.

Mercury Toxicity

Hg Intake per Source:

Dental amalgam filling (Hg vapor): according to the American Dental Association: 1.0–2.0 mcg/day

Dental amalgam filling (Hg vapor): according to the World Health Organization: 3.0–17.5 mcg/day (average 10 mcg/day, extreme 100 mcg/day)

Fish 2.4 mcg/day

Non-fish food: 0.3 mcg/day

Air, water, food: 3.09 mcg/day

Miscellaneous

Chronic fatigue, frequent urination, bloated feeling after eating, recurring constipation, ringing in the ears, metallic taste in mouth, TMJ, headaches after eating, hormonal irregularities, low sex drive, suicidal thoughts, airborne allergies, food allergies, severe digestive problems including Candida, Crohn's, and other digestive flora-related illnesses. Mercury toxic individuals may excrete mercury via sweat, saliva, feces, urine, and semen. Mercury can move freely through fetal blood supplies and breast milk, causing potential danger to unborn and nursing children.

With such a large variety of painful and debilitating conditions associated with mercury, clearly there is no such thing as a "safe amount" of this metal in your body. Because of mercury's unique ability to be transmitted through the generations, this toxic metal will continue on with its destructive work in a perpetual manner until people realize that many of their current health problems are actually mercury related. Cleaning the human system of this poisonous substance should be a top priority for anyone interested in good health.

As was mentioned earlier, the hair analysis is a great way to assess the human body's toxic burden because this diagnostic tool measures long-term toxic levels. Some toxins are quickly removed from the blood and urine because the body simply cannot tolerate them. If the toxins cannot be excreted quickly, the body resorts to hiding the toxins in fat and tissues. This is one reason why blood and urine samples are notoriously inaccurate for mercury toxicity. This unfortunately gives people who are truly mercury toxic a false sense of security.

One caveat that needs to be mentioned is that while the hair analysis is a fantastic diagnostic tool, it does not *directly* measure the body's mercury burden. My baseline data showed a relatively low level of mercury, though without a doubt my levels were extremely high. The real value in the hair analysis is its measurement of the other toxins in the body. Dr. Andrew Cutler wrote an entire book on how to utilize hair analysis reports to diagnose mercury toxicity. While this book is useful (and it is shown in the Reference section), I don't believe it is required reading for most people. Mercury metal is a type of linchpin for most of the other toxic metals. Once you get rid of the mercury linchpin, the other toxins are rapidly excreted. It all centers on mercury. I detoxed myself using the various protocols in this book. As I detoxed, I excreted large volumes of mercury. This caused the other toxins in my body to drop, and these metal reductions were clearly shown in the hair analysis reports.

The Doctor's Data Hair Analysis can be ordered through Dr. Alan Greenberg's very helpful website: www.scienceformulas.com. This was also the site where

I ordered many of my chelation supplements as well as some multivitamin supplements. Hair analysis kits can also be found online (www.amazon.com) or directly through laboratories (www.testcountry.com).

Depending on where you live, getting lab work done easily, quickly, and inexpensively can be difficult. I found working through www.requestatest.com for lab tests to be a great way to get data without the trouble or expense of a doctor's office visit. You order a test online, and then show up at a local clinic a few days later with a confirmation letter and code. A lab worker takes a blood sample, and you get your results within 1-2 weeks.

Chapter 2: Stopping the Source

You can find a biological dentist at http://holisticdental.org/find-a-holistic-dentist.

My dentist is found here, and I highly recommend this type of dentistry for mercury removal because these dentists use several important precautionary steps. Prior to my amalgam filling removal, I was given activated charcoal. During the extraction process, I was given protective eyewear, oxygen gas, and suction was used throughout my time in the chair. Also, a large rubber dam was inserted in my mouth to collect any larger pieces of mercury. These were all used in conjunction so that any reintroduction of mercury into my system was greatly minimized. This dentist was also the one who removed my four root canal implants. Four missing teeth is no laughing matter, literally, and so I was fitted with a flesh-colored plastic retainer with four false teeth. This retainer fits neatly into my mouth and is nearly impossible to detect by others. The retainer allows me to smile broadly, laugh out loud, and chew any type of food with no issues whatsoever.

There are a large number of very fine water treatment systems available that can reduce or remove your exposure to toxins in tap water. With so many good systems available, the real question centers around how much you are willing to spend. Two extremely inexpensive in-shower systems we have used are from Sprite, www.spritewater.com/, and from Aquasana, www.aquasana.com/. Aquasana also offers a whole-home system which we have used for years with great results.

Chapter 3: The Quickest Cleanse

There are some powerful preventative measures you can take to reduce the frequency and severity of kidney stone attacks. Of course, doing regular kidney cleanses are a great first step, but in order to keep the stones from returning, you need to do more. I have found that taking a high quality magnesium supplement is vital for preventing kidney stones from returning. If you look into the research on magnesium absorption rates, you will probably find what I did years ago: many if not most nutritional supplements are almost worthless. The supplement magnesium oxide is a great example of what I mean. Of all of the magnesium supplements available, magnesium oxide is perhaps the most commonly one found in a typical multivitamin. It is also the most poorly absorbed form of magnesium. The reason it is in so many multivitamins is because it is so inexpensive, and supplement manufacturers want to advertise a product that contains magnesium. *Sigh.*

I recommend doing your research to find the best, most highly absorbed magnesium supplement. If you do the research, you will probably find what I found: magnesium malate is one of the best forms available. I have used magnesium citrate with good results, but I have found the best results with magnesium malate. Since magnesium is at the center of nearly 300 human body enzymatic reactions, it is a great idea to take a full dose of magnesium daily.

Taking a high quality Vitamin C is also strongly recommended. Take 2-4 grams of this daily, if you can tolerate it. (Yes, you read this correctly—grams). To avoid diarrhea, this may take some time to work up to gram amounts. But over the course of several months, this is easily achieved. If you do your research, you will find that what exists for magnesium is also true with Vitamin C. Not all Vitamin C is created equally. Actually, it probably was created equally in the very beginning, but food quality and nutrient quality has been slowly diminishing ever since. Much, if not most of the Vitamin C produced in the US today is from corn. Much if not most of this corn has had its genetic backbone tampered with by genetic engineers. Many suspect that this is the reason why so much Vitamin C on the market today is nearly worthless. The goal is to get Vitamin C from a non-corn based source that is also non-GMO (genetically modified organism). Two non-corn based Vitamin C sources that I have found to be excellent are Super-C Option from BioImmune and Vitamin C from Ecological Formulas.

Drinking at least 1-2 liters of filtered or distilled water daily is also recommended for keeping your kidneys clean and clear. *I know what you are thinking.* 1-2 liters does seem like a great deal of water. But when you read the research on how most people today are walking around in a slightly dehydrated state, 1-2 liters of water seems quite reasonable. And no, drinking juice or milk or any other drink other than distilled or filtered water does not count. Try to avoid drinking water that has been treated with chlorine or fluoride. Unfortunately, this includes most if not all water sources from the municipal water supply. However, fluoride and chlorine are powerful chemicals. Even in trace amounts, these halides cause the body to excrete iodine, and are therefore harmful to all four of the filters you are trying to clean.

Chapter 4: The Misunderstood Cleanse

Finding high quality supplements is not easy. There are too many companies that exist today mainly because of a lack of education on the part of the consumer. Far too often I wasted money on nutritional supplements that were useless. I trusted these companies to provide me with high quality supplements. I needed high quality supplements to help me regain my lost health. Unfortunately, this was simply blind trust. Once I began doing research into the actual ingredients in supplements, I became much more discriminating with my purchases. It is important that you learn to distinguish between high and low quality supplements, because supplements that truly are of high quality can bring a person a long way towards great health. But of course, not everyone can do extensive research on their supplements. A certain amount of trust is required. This is unavoidable. Having said as much, I found the *Multi Chelation Support Formula* to be an excellent choice for a multivitamin. This supplement is available from www.scienceformulas.com. Another excellent choice for a multivitamin is the Multigenics Intensive Care from Metagenics. This can be purchased through Amazon. With both of these multivitamins, I recommend taking the dosage as noted on the bottle.

For iodine supplementation, I used at various times Iodoral, Nascent iodine, and Lugal's 2% and 5% iodine solution. Iodoral and Lugal's are essentially the same type of iodine, which is a mixture of iodine in elemental (iodine) form and molecular (iodide) form. The human body utilizes both of these forms of iodine, and this is the iodine type recommended in the *12 Step Detox*. If you are interested in looking into the iodine issue in greater detail, Stephanie Burst's excellent paper on the subject, ("Guide to Supplementing with Iodine) can be found here: http://jeffreydachmd.com/wp-content/uploads/2014/03/The-Guide-to-Supplementing-with-Iodine-Stephanie-Burst-ND.pdf

If you are taking Vitamin C during the thyroid cleanse, make sure you take the Vitamin C several hours before or after the iodine. These two supplements have a canceling effect on each other, and several hours is required in order to avoid this conflict.

Chapter 5: The Dreaded Liver Flush

The liver flush is a very powerful detox protocol. However, there are some aspects of this protocol that are problematic. After doing several flushes, I found a few solutions to some of the more notorious problems associated with the liver flush. The first problem is drinking all of that apple cider. I have already shared an easy solution to this. Instead of drinking the cider, take 1 gram of malic acid per day for two weeks. The second dilemma is the taking of Epsom salts. This type of salt tastes very bitter and it makes any drink taste terrible.

You can find Epsom salts (magnesium sulfate) in pill form on the Web. Many people find taking magnesium sulfate pills to be far easier than drinking down a tablespoon of this chemical mixed with water or juice. The third dilemma of the liver flush is drinking a ½ cup of oil. The good news with the oil is that this amount of oil may be flexible. I have done successful liver flushes with only a ¼ cup of oil. Yes, a ¼ cup of oil is still a significant amount of oil, but it beats drinking ½ of a cup of oil! Also, there is nothing wrong with trying to improve the taste of the olive oil. You can mix the olive oil with some coconut oil to improve the taste. It's a helpful way to get the oil down, and to stay down.

A final problem of the liver flush is the terrible nausea that often follows the flush itself. Sometimes I could do a liver flush with absolutely no problems whatsoever. At other times, I felt like I was hit by a train. As a remedy for the nausea, I take activated charcoal immediately after I drink my oil. Liver flushes release a tremendous amount of pent up bile all at once. This bile goes through the intestines in volumes that the body may not have experienced in years. Bile kills harmful microorganisms living in the intestines and these tiny critters spill their toxins into the body as they die. The bile also carries toxins out of the body, and some of these toxins make their way back into the bloodstream. The bottom line is that a liver flush may release a tremendous amount of toxic waste that was stored up in the body. The activated charcoal can neutralize much of this toxic waste and the result is that you may feel less nausea as you are going through the process. Taking a few grams of activated charcoal immediately after ingesting the oil may remove much of the nausea that a liver flush sometimes inflicts.

Chapter 6: Preparing for a Healing Crisis

One additional technique that I found very useful in minimizing the effects of a healing crisis is vigorous exercise. But getting on the stationary bicycle or treadmill is often the last thing you feel like doing when you begin to experience a healing crisis. Also, the timing usually is very inconvenient. As has already been mentioned, when I would be going through a healing crisis, I often broke out in hives and swelling. This usually occurred at night. Far too many times to count, I would feel my face begin to swell up around bedtime. This forced me to make a choice. Go to bed and wake up in the morning very red and swollen, or stay up for hours and get on the treadmill until the healing crisis passed. Neither choice was desirable, but I usually would get on that treadmill because the hives and swelling were simply too painful to deal with.

In terms of activated charcoal and probiotics, I have found that using the medical grade quality is the best you can have. I prefer the Norit A Supra USP from www.buyactivatedcharcoal.com to be the best value for the money. For the probiotics, I have not found any product that even comes close to VSL #3, available online at http://www.vsl3.com/hcp/faq/. It can also be purchased at Costco in the pharmacy section. VSL #3, like the Norit A Supra, are medical grade supplements that I have found to be amazingly effective. The recommended dosage on the VSL#3 bottle is broad, 3-8 capsules per day. As with most supplements, I suggest starting on the low end and slowly working upwards.

One special technique I have found to be very useful with increasing the effectiveness of the VSL #3 is to place the probiotic capsule into an empty capsule. The VSL #3 comes in 00 sized capsules. I take these and place them in empty 000 sized capsules. Most people need probiotics, but far too often the probiotic capsule opens in the stomach and the probiotics are exposed to hydrochloric acid. This acid destroys most of the living bacteria. The stomach can't be blamed for this. It is only doing what it was designed to do: kill living things. A typical probiotic capsule lasts for about 5 minutes in an acid solution. This is true even for an enteric coated capsule. By doubling my capsules, I double my time of transit. This gives the probiotic about 10 minutes to pass through the stomach and reach the small intestines, where it then opens and floods the area with healthy bacteria.

Chapter 7: The Intestinal Cleanse

Of all the detox protocols available, I have found that food grade diatomaceous earth (DE) is one of the best kept secrets around. It is an amazing supplement.

Unfortunately, few people seem to be talking about DE, and even fewer are taking it. Food grade DE has been used as a powerful anti-parasitic for farm livestock for years. But why should only the pigs and cows be parasite-free? DE is incredibly powerful, safe, and extremely cost-effective. You can buy it in bulk by the pound for around six dollars. I recommend the DE by Earthworks Health at http://www.earthworkshealth.com/human-use.php. This website also contains a great deal of useful information that anyone who is considering doing an intestinal detox should consider. Two cautions with DE. First, begin slowly and work up your dosages. I began with just a teaspoon or so and worked my way up to three or four heaping tablespoons. You know you are getting good results from the DE when you see a rather substantial increase in the amount of daily solid waste you produce. Simply judging from the putrid and pungent smell of the solid waste, you know something nasty has been eliminated. The second caution is to avoid inhaling the DE. It is a very light powder and quickly becomes airborne if not handled properly. I place it immediately in warm water, stir it in slowly, and then add my juices for a better tasting DE smoothie.

As has already been mentioned, I used VSL #3 for my intestinal cleanse and have found it to be superior to any other probiotic on the market today. For the anti-fungal aspect of the intestinal cleanse, I found Garden of Life's *Fungal Defense* and *Raw Candida Cleanse* to be excellent supplements. After doing a significant amount of research on human parasites, I decided it was best to play it safe and not assume I was entirely free from any intestinal bugs. I used Humaworm's proprietary product, *Humaworm*, for several months. I never found any evidence of anything in my feces, but then again, I couldn't get myself to look for them either. I think this is an outstanding product, and the website, https://humaworm.com/ is full of great information.

If you choose to add the option essential oils protocol to your intestinal cleanse, you will need to do a bit of experimentation. I have found working with essential oils to be extremely helpful, but also a bit challenging. The first challenge is simply to be able to find high quality oils. There are a plethora of essential oil brands on the market, but I have found very few that really could deliver on their promises. A good example of this is with oil of oregano. This is an extremely potent oil, but there are many "junk oregano oils" on the market that are too weak to do any good. To my knowledge, the only type of oregano oil that has the powerful antibacterial, antifungal qualities is the *Origanum vulgare* variety.

In a similar manner, the thyme oil of the vulgaris variety has strong antifungal abilities, and this is the brand that I used with great success in my experimentation with essential oils. But even when you get the right plant species, you may find that the oil is seriously diluted. After a significant amount of trial and error, I found a super strong oil of oregano on Amazon at http://www.amazon.com/Oregano-Strenght-Carvacol-Pharmaceutical-Mountains/dp/B005GJTO9S. Since this oil is not diluted, you need to dilute it to suit your own tastes. It is far too strong for direct contact with the skin and it *will* cause a chemical burn very quickly. I dilute this oil with either olive, coconut, castor oil, or avocado oil. I also have experimented with mixing various oils with strong anti-fungal, anti-bacterial, and anti-viral properties. These oils include clove, cinnamon, lemon, peppermint, and licorice oils. I have mixed these in various ratios with the thyme and oregano oils and received excellent results.

Chapter 8: Chelation

There are several good products on the market that can be used for effective chelation.

Two products that I have used over the years are *Chelorex*, from Science Formulas, and *Detox Max Plus* from BioImmune. Here are two sites that offer these products:

http://www.scienceformulas.com/how.html

http://www.agriorganics.com/natural.php?Pid=3

I prefer these products for different reasons. Chelorex utilizes high quality ingredients that work synergistically, and it utilizes the best excretion pathway—the intestines. From all I found in the research, chelating heavy metals like mercury should be done using the intestines and not the kidneys due to their high sensitivity and potential for damage when excreting large amounts of heavy metals. Detox Max Plus does utilize the kidneys, but because it is a slow-release chelating compound, the amount of irritation and inflammation that may occur in the kidneys is greatly minimized. Detox Max Plus also has the huge advantage of being available in a liquid form, which is almost essential when chelating small children.

Chapter 9: Dietary Changes and Challenges

Of all the changes I experienced when I first began to detox successfully, the change in food desires was certainly one of the most surprising. Looking back, it all makes complete sense now. A newly cleaned up intestinal network would be able to communicate more effectively with the rest of the body. Now that my digestive system was cleaned up, it was communicating to my brain more effectively (and vice versa) concerning exactly what is, and what is not, good food. If this is how the internal system works regarding food, I began to see junk food as far more dangerous than what I previously thought. Junk food is loaded with toxic chemicals, including dyes, flavor enhancers, and synthetic chemicals. Over time, these toxins accumulate within the body and dulls a person's ability to make good food choices. Once I started to get cleaned up, food took on a whole new level of meaning for me. My food desires were truly transformed. I loved this change in food desires. This made the detox experience so much more powerful. It was more than just correcting problems from the past. Detoxing was now making for a better future. This also increased my will power. Saying *no* to cookies loaded with high fructose corn syrup and MSG was so much easier now. I knew in my mind that these "foods" were bad, and now my body was gradually losing its desire for these substances as well. This was not only a strong indicator that the detox was working, it was great for building my confidence and willpower going forward in life. I was gradually becoming stronger and healthier, and I was doing it in ways that were truly gratifying. Detoxing had become more than just a necessity. It became a true labor of joy because it was transforming me into a far better person than what I had been before.

Chapter 10: Exercise and Rest

There is a very simple relationship between physical activity and toxicity. As you increase in toxicity, you will decrease in physical activity. The limiting factor in this relationship is inflammation.

Toxins place a great deal of stress on a biological system. This stress causes internal inflammation to increase. This in turn reduces your range of physical abilities. Detoxing reduces this inflammation because it removes the chemicals that are causing the inflammation in the first place. Speaking personally, this reduction in inflammation caused several weird and inexplicable health problems to simply vanish. This may sound strange, but it makes perfect sense. Take out poisons that are causing health problems and inflammation, and your body can build and repair itself. This rebuilding was demonstrated most dramatically with my testosterone level.

As my internal inflammation began to decrease, cortisol production also decreased causing testosterone levels to increase. *I was actually increasing testosterone levels in an all-natural manner! Yes!* The testosterone boost gave me plenty of extra energy, and this extra energy allowed me to get back into the gym in a big way. I used to be really into body-building, and *Detox Memoir* contains some interesting stories concerning this area of my past. But now things were different. I was obviously older, but now I found that I could bulk up much more quickly than ever before. Though I am sure I would have thought differently about this 20 years earlier, I had little interest now with "getting huge." These days, I just wanted to stay fit. And staying fit was very easy to do after I had detoxed. My body was far more responsive to exercise, food, and sleep. I had improved in all of these areas. A small amount of exercise on a daily basis yielded fantastic results. My food requirements were less than what they used to be, and foods even tasted better. Furthermore, if I did get an injury— usually sports related—I healed more quickly than I had before. Finally, my sleep had improved as well. I needed less sleep, and as far as I could tell, I slept more soundly.

Chapter 11: Pacing

Pacing your own detox is an individual thing that must be done carefully. If you are planning on cleaning out the four filter areas of your body, how much protocol-overlap are you willing to try during your detox? This is a very good question that each person must consider. Listening to your body, and keeping a vigilant eye out for the sometimes sneaky healing crisis should be top priorities. I say this in full confidence now. However, when I was first learning how to detox properly, I would go for several months knowing full well that my pacing and dosage levels were too high for my body to tolerate. These actions would invariably invoke a healing crisis. I knew this in advance, but I did it anyway. I wanted to finish my detox and I decided the pain and suffering was worth the almost constant healing crisis. Looking back, I wish I would have learned sooner about implementing those key steps that can effectively alleviate a healing crisis. Using activated charcoal more regularly would have been at the top of my list. Once I did learn about activated charcoal, I used it faithfully nearly every day for many months to keep the hives and swelling away. Over time as my body healed, taking activated charcoal became far less frequent as it was no longer necessary.

Keeping a journal and constantly updating it is a very good idea for anyone who is detoxing. A journal can also help you set the proper pacing for your detox. This is particularly important if you wish to overlap the protocols. There are so many important variables that are in play when detoxing. Recording dosages, dates, times, and responses to various protocols is truly essential. This data will serve as an excellent guide as you move forward with your detox. The journal will also be a source of great encouragement as you see progress in your health. You are essentially creating your own "before" and "after" picture of yourself with your journaling. With every little victory, you will find added motivation to continue with your detox until you reach a level of health that is truly satisfying.

Chapter 12: Reflection

Doing ongoing maintenance-level detox protocols is an excellent way to keep your health at a very high level. I still take my high quality multivitamins daily. I do a thyroid tune up using iodine, selenium, and zinc once a year or so, and I try to do a liver flush twice a year. I also do an intestinal cleanse with food grade diatomaceous earth periodically to keep the intestines clean and clear. I have found that the benefits gained from using these detox protocols for routine maintenance far outweighs any inconvenience experienced by doing them. I have especially found a tremendous amount of benefit from doing regular kidney cleanses. These are quick, easy, and powerfully effective.

Acknowledgments

would like to thank several people for assisting with the content and writing of this book. First a special thanks to my loving and patient family members who provided me with encouragement, advice, and at times, data from their own detoxes. I would like to say thank you to my reader-editors: Mary Ann Rivers, Jill Gregory, and Deirdre Kermis for their thoughtful insight and encouragement. Special thanks to my amazing editor Kevin Ashby Whitted, who always brings the quality of my writing up more than just a few notches. Finally, I'd like to say thanks to my good friends Dr. Kevin Wall and Mr. Doug Fougnies, who gave me the idea to write this book in the first place.

References

Chapter 1: A History of Toxicity

American Dental Association Council on Scientific Affairs (2010). Literature review: dental amalgam fillings and health effects. Retrieved from http://www.ada.org/en/member-center/oral-health-topics/amalgam

Cutler, A. (1999). *Hair Test Interpretation: Finding Hidden Toxicities*. Noamalgam.com.

Haley, B. (2005). Mercury toxicity: genetic susceptibility, and synergistic effects. *Medical Veritas*, 2:535–542. Retrieved from http://homeoint.ru/pdfs/haley.pdf

Huggins, H. (1993). *It's All in Your Head—The Link Between Mercury Amalgam and Illness*. New York, NY: Penguin Putnam.

Kennedy, D. (2011). US FDA hearings on amalgam safety. Retrieved from https://www.youtube.com/watch?v=jK2Uy49Z6CA and https://www.youtube.com/watch?v=pUcSrOycSME

Koral, Stephen M., (2005). The scientific case against amalgam. *International Academy of Oral Medicine & Toxicology.* Retrieved from http://iaomt.org/wp-content/uploads/The-Case-Against-Amalgam.pdf

Levy, T. & Huggins, H. (1999). *Uniformed Consent—The Hidden Dangers in Dental Care.* Newburyport, MS: Hampton Publishing.

Siegel, S., Stratton, L., Bender, B., & Gutierrez, R. (2003) Mercury exposé: the world's toxic time bomb. Prepared for the 22nd United Nations Environment Programme, Nairobi. Retrieved from http://www.ban.org/Ban-Hg-Wg/Mercury.ToxicTimeBomb.Final.PDF

Windham, B. (2001). Mercury exposure levels from amalgam dental fillings; documentation of mechanisms by which mercury causes over 40 chronic health conditions; results of replacement of amalgam fillings; and occupational effects on dental staff. Retrieved from http://www.fda.gov/ohrms/dockets/dailys/02/Sep02/091602/80027dde.pdf

United States Department of Health and Human Services (1999). Public Health Statement: Mercury. Cas#: 7439-97-6. Washington D.C. Government Printing Office. Retrieved from http://www.atsdr.cdc.gov/ToxProfiles/tp46-c1-b.pdf

United States Environmental Protection Agency (1997). Mercury study report to Congress vol. 5: health effects of mercury and mercury compounds. Washington D.C. Government Printing Office. Retrieved from http://www.epa.gov/ttn/oarpg/t3/reports/volume5.pdf

United States Environmental Protection Agency (2013). Mercury in dental amalgam. Retrieved from http://www.epa.gov/hg/dentalamalgam.html

United States Food and Drug Administration (2009). Dental devices: classification of dental amalgam, reclassification of dental mercury, designation of special controls for dental amalgam, mercury, and amalgam alloy. Food and Drug Administration, Dept. of Health and Human Services. Retrieved from http://www.fda.gov/downloads/medicaldevices/productsandmedicalprocedures/dentalproducts/dentalamalgam/ucm174024.pdf

Chapter 2: Stopping the Source

American Environmental Health Studies Project (2004). *The Fluoride Deception.* Retrieved from https://www.youtube.com/watch?v=eBZRb-73tLc

Bryson, C. (2004). *The Fluoride Deception.* New York, NY: Seven Stories Press.

Cann, S., van Netten, J., & van Netten, C. (2000). Hypothesis: iodine, selenium, and the development of breast cancer. *Cancer Causes and Control,* 11:121–127. Retrieved from http://link.springer.com/article/10.1023/A:1008925301459#page-1

Cutler, A. (1999). *Amalgam Illness, Diagnosis and Treatment: What You Can Do to Get Better, How Your Doctor Can Help.* Sammamish, WA: Andrew Hall Cutler Publishing.

Dush, D. (2001). Breast implants and illness: a model of psychological factors. *Annals of the Rheumatic Diseases.* **60**:653-657 doi:10.1136/ard.60.7.653. Retrieved from http://ard.bmj.com/content/60/7/653.full

Fisk, M., et al. (2010). Asthma in swimmers: a review of the current literature. *The Physician and Sports Medicine.* 38(4):28–34. Retrieved from http://www.ncbi.nlm.nih.gov/pubmed/21150139

Institute for Agriculture and Trade Policy. (2009, Jan. 28). Study finds high-fructose corn syrup contains mercury. *The Washington Post.* Retrieved from http://www.washingtonpost.com/wp-dyn/content/article/2009/01/26/AR2009012601831.html

Kolb, S. (20090. *The Naked Truth About Breast Implants: From Harm to Healing.* Minnesota. Lighthouse Publishing.

Mercola, J. (2012). The naked truth about breast implants—how they can affect your health. November 12. Retrieved from http://articles.mercola.com/sites/articles/archive/2012/11/18/dr-kolb-discusses-breast-implants.aspx

Price, W. (1923). *Dental Infections, Oral and Systemic*, Vol. I, Penton Pub Co. Ohio, USA.

Saray, A., et al. (2004). Some effects of lead contamination on liver and gallbladder bile. *Plastic and Reconstructive Surgery*, Oct., 114(5): 1170-8. Retrieved from http://www.ncbi.nlm.nih.gov/pubmed/15457030

Sharp, D. (2002). Silicone breast implants: correlation between implant ruptures, magnetic resonance spectroscopically estimated silicone presence in the liver, antibody status and clinical symptoms. *Rheumatology.* 41:123-124 doi:10.1093/rheumatology/41.2.123. Retrieved from http://rheumatology.oxfordjournals.org/content/41/2/123.full.pdf+html

Chapter 3: The Quickest Cleanse

Hering, F., et al. (1985). Fluoridation of drinking water: effects on kidney stone formation. *Urological Research*, 13(4): 175-178. Retrieved from http://www.ncbi.nlm.nih.gov/pubmed/4049603

Howenstein, J. (2008 Apr.12). Parsley tea for urinary tract infections and kidney stones. *NewsWithViews.com.* Retrieved from http://www.newswithviews.com/Howenstine/james65.htm

Kurland, E., et al. (2007). Recovery from skeletal fluorosis. *Journal of Bone and Mineral Research*, 22(1): 163-170. Retrieved from http://onlinelibrary.wiley.com/doi/10.1359/jbmr.060912/epdf

Ludlow, M., et al. (2007). Effects of fluoridation of community water supplies for people with chronic kidney disease. *Nephrology Dialysis Transplantation*, 22: 2763-2767. doi:10.1093/ndt/gfm477. Retrieved from https://www.kidney.org/sites/default/files/docs/khafluoridation_ckd-ndt_2007.pdf

Chapter 4: The Misunderstood Cleanse

Abraham, G. (2005). The historical background of the iodine project. *The Original Internist*. Summer: 57–66. Retrieved from http://www.optimox.com/pics/Iodine/pdfs/IOD08.pdf

Brownstein, D. (2005). Orthosupplementation. *The Original Internist*. 12(3):105–108. Retrieved from http://iodineresearch.com/orthobrownstien.html

Brownstein, D. (2008). *Overcoming Thyroid Disorders*. (3rd ed.). West Bloomfield, MI: Medical Alternative Press.

Brownstein, D. (2009). *Iodine: Why You Need It, Why You Can't Live without It*. (4th ed.). West Bloomfield, MI: Medical Alternative Press.

Ertek, S., Cicero, A., Caglar, O., & Erdogan, G. (2010). Relationship between serum zinc levels, thyroid hormones and thyroid volume following successful iodine supplementation. *Hormones* 9(3):263–268. Retrieved from http://www.hormones.gr/pdf/HORMONES%202010%20263-268.pdf

Feldkamp, J., et al. (1999). Fas-mediated apoptosis is inhibited by TSH and iodine in moderate concentrations in primary human thyrocytes in vitro. *Hormone and Metabolic Research*, 31(6):355–358. Retrieved from https://www.thieme-connect.com/products/ejournals/abstract/10.1055/s-2007-978753

Goldman, M. & Blackburn, P. (1979). The effect of mercuric chloride on thyroid function in the rat. *Toxicology and Applied Pharmacology* 48(1):49–55. Retrieved from http://www.sciencedirect.com/science/article/pii/S0041008X79800071

Köhrle, J., Oertel, M. & Gross, M. (1992). Selenium supply regulates thyroid function, thyroid hormone synthesis and metabolism by altering the expression of selenoenzymes Type I 5'-deiodinase and glutathione peroxidase. *Thyridology* 4(1):17–21. Retrieved from http://www.ncbi.nlm.nih.gov/pubmed/1284327

Köhrle, J. (2000). The deiodinase family: selenoenzymes regulating thyroid hormone availability and action. *Cellular and Molecular Life Sciences* 57(13–14): 1853–1863. Retrieved from http://www.ncbi.nlm.nih.gov/pubmed/11215512

Lauritano, E., et al. (2007). Association between hypothyroidism and small intestinal bacterial overgrowth. *The Journal of Endocrinology and Metabolism*, Nov; 92(11): 4180-4184. Retrieved from http://www.ncbi.nlm.nih.gov/pubmed/17698907/

Mercola, J. (2009). Avoid this if you want to keep your thyroid healthy. Retrieved from http://articles.mercola.com/sites/articles/archive/2009/09/05/Another-Poison-Hiding-in-Your-Environment.aspx

Patrick, L. (2008). Iodine: deficiency and therapeutic considerations. *Alternative Medicine Review*, 13(2):116–127. Retrieved from http://web.a.ebscohost.com/abstract?direct=true&profile=ehost&scope=site&authtype=crawler&jrnl=10895159&AN=33337826&h=6PjaZtsF04kxnLvXiKMOIvA2JdbPL3998uLm2t8%2fJQinGknfiOTXjtsMjKptuMKPICMUhBDsSBov7MKFKni2zA%3d%3d&crl=c

Piccone, N. (2011). The silent epidemic of iodine deficiency. *Life Extension Magazine*, October. Retrieved from http://www.lef.org/magazine/mag2011/oct2011_The-Silent-Epidemic-of-Iodine-Deficiency_01.htm

Power, L. (2006). Iodine & thyroid deficiencies: linked to thyroid and breast cancer, fibrocystic breast disease, infertility, obesity, mental retardation & halide toxemia. Retrieved from http://www.laurapower.com/page26.html

Sircus, M. (2011). Iodine phobia & salt truth. *International Veritas Medical Association.* Retrieved from http://drsircus.com/medicine/iodine/iodine-phobia-salt-truth#_ednref2

Sugiura, Y., Tamai, Y., & Tanaka, H. (1978). Selenium protection against mercury toxicity: high binding affinity of methylmercury by selenium-containing ligands in comparison with sulfur-containing ligands. *Bioinorganic Chemistry* 9(2): 167–180. Retrieved from http://www.sciencedirect.com/science/article/pii/S0006306100802884

Vassilakis, J. & Nicolopoulos, N. (1981). Dissolution of gallstones following thyroxine administration. A case report. *Hepato-gastroenterology,* 28(1):60–61. Retrieved from http://europepmc.org/abstract/MED/6894289/reload=0;jsessionid=dmGG5UKUxWDyUrOezjIk.12

Völzke, H., Robinson, D., & Ulrich, J. (2005). Association between thyroid function and gallstone disease. *World Journal of Gastroenterology* 11(35):5530–5534. Retrieved from http://www.wjgnet.com/1007-9327/11/5530.pdf?origin=publication_detail

World Health Organization (2007). Iodine deficiency in Europe: A continuing public health problem. *WHO.* Retrieved from http://www.who.int/nutrition/publications/VMNIS_Iodine_deficiency_in_Europe.pdf

Wu, P. (2000). Thyroid disease and diabetes. *Clinical Diabetes* 18(1). Retrieved from http://journal.diabetes.org/clinicaldiabetes/v18n12000/pg38.htm

Chapter 5: The Dreaded Liver Flush

Brody, J. (1995, May 31). Personal health; gallbladder surgery is easier. Is it too common? *The New York Times.* Retrieved from http://www.nytimes.com/1995/05/31/us/personal-health-gallbladder-surgery-is-easier-is-it-too-common.html

Georgiou, G. (2007). Flushing gallstones naturally. Retrieved from http://www.collegenaturalmedicine.com/images/LBA/liver%20cleansing%202007.pdf

Howenstein, J. (2007 Dec.3). Bile salts can heal psoriasis, septicemia, viral infections, and excess estrogen. *NewsWithViews.com*. Retrieved from http://www.newswithviews.com/Howenstine/james63.htm

Johns Hopkins Medicine (2001). Gallstone disease: introduction. Retrieved from http://www.hopkinsmedicine.org/gastroenterology_hepatology/_pdfs/pancreas_biliary_tract/gallstone_disease.pdf

Méndez-Sánchez, N., et al. (2005). Metabolic syndrome as a risk factor for gallstone disease. *World Journal of Gastroenterology* 11, 1653–1657.

Moritz, A. (2007). *The Liver and Gallbladder Miracle Cleanse: An All-Natural, At-Home Flush to Purify and Rejuvenate Your Body*. Ener-chi.com: North Carolina.

Srisukho, S., et al. (1996). Mercury content in the gallstones and bile of Thai people (Chiang Mai and Bangkok) and Japanese. *Journal of the Medical Association of Thailand*, 79(5), 299-308. Retrieved from http://www.ncbi.nlm.nih.gov/pubmed/8708522

Chapter 6: Preparing for a Healing Crisis

Absar, A., et al. (2010). The global war against intestinal parasites—should we use a holistic approach? *International Journal of Infectious Diseases*. 14:732–738. doi:10.1016/j.ijid.2009.11.036

Berger, J., Redinger, R., & Small, D. (1970). Instrument for sampling and measuring bile flow. *Medical & Biological Engineering & Computing*. 8(1):19–24. Retrieved from http://link.springer.com/article/10.1007%2FBF02551745

Boroch, A. (2008). *The Candida Cure. Yeast, Fungus, & Your Health*. Los Angeles, CA: Quintessential Healing Publishing, Inc.

Clark, H. (1996). How parasites causes cancer and HIV. *The Light Party*. Retrieved from http://www.lightparty.com/Health/PARASITE.html

Cook, G. (1994). Enterobius vermicularis infection. *GUT*. 35(9):1159–1162. Retrieved from http://www.ncbi.nlm.nih.gov/pmc/articles/PMC1375686/

Crompton, D. (1984). *Parasites and people*. London, England. Macmillan Publishers, Ltd.

Crompton, D. & Savioli, L. (1993). Intestinal parasitic infections and urbanization. *Bulletin of the World Health Organization*. 71(1):1–7. Retrieved from http://apps.who.int/iris/handle/10665/49956

Dinsley, J. (2006). *Charcoal Remedies.Com. The Complete Handbook of Medicinal Charcoal and Its Applications*. GateKeepers Book.

Ehrlich, S. (2012). Internal parasites. *Complementary and Alternative Medicine Guide, University of Maryland Medical Center*. Retrieved from http://umm.edu/health/medical/altmed/condition/intestinal-parasites

Mercola, J. & Klinghardt, D. (2001). Mercury toxicity and systemic elimination agents. *Journal of Nutritional & Environmental Medicine*. (11):53–62. Retrieved from http://www.biblelife.org/Mercury-toxicity-Dr-Klinghardt.pdf

Murray, A. & Kidby, D. (1975). Subcellular location of mercury in yeast grown in the presence of mercuric chloride. *Journal of General Microbiology*. (86):66–74. Retrieved from http://mic.sgmjournals.org/content/86/1/66.full.pdf+html

Chapter 7: The Intestinal Cleanse

Akdemir, E. (2015). Empirical prediction and validation of antibacterial inhibitory effects of various plant essential oils. *International Journal of Food Microbiology*. Jun. 2; 202: 35-41. doi: 10.1016/j.ijfoodmicro.2015.02.030. Retrieved from http://www.ncbi.nlm.nih.gov/pubmed/25764982

Aldenborg, F., Fall, M, & Enerback, L. (1986). Proliferation and transepithelial migration of mucosal mast cells in interstitial cystitis. *Immunology*. 58:411–416. Retrieved from http://www.ncbi.nlm.nih.gov/pmc/articles/PMC1453481/

Basuroy, S., et al. (2005). Acetaldehyde disrupts tight junctions and adherens junctions in human colonic mucosa: protection by EGF and L-glutamine. *American Journal of Physiology*. Aug; 289(2): G367-75. Retrieved from http://www.ncbi.nlm.nih.gov/pubmed/15718285

Bennett D., et al. (2011). Effect of diatomaceous earth on parasite load, egg production, and egg quality of free-range organic laying hens. *Poultry Science*. July; 90(7):1416-26. doi: 10.3382/ps.2010-01256. Retrieved from http://www.ncbi.nlm.nih.gov/pubmed/21673156

Bethony, J., et al. (2006). Soil-transmitted helminth infections: ascariasis, trichuriasis, and hookworm. *The Lance.com*. May 6. 367:1521–1532. Retrieved from http://140.226.65.22/Davis_lab/Parasit_links/Soil_Transmitted_%20 Helminths_Lancet_%20'06.pdf

Danil de Namor A., et. al. (2012). Turning the volume down on heavy metals using tuned diatomite. A review of diatomite and modified diatomite for the extraction of heavy metals from water. *Journal of Hazardous Materials*. November 30; 241-242:14-31. doi: 10.1016/j.jhazmat.2012.09.030. Retrieved from http://www.ncbi.nlm.nih.gov/pubmed/23062514

Duval-Araujo, I., et al. (2007). Bacterial colonization of the ileum in rats with obstructive jaundice. *Brazilian Journal of Microbiology*. 38:406–408. Retrieved from http://www.scielo.br/scielo.php?pid=S1517-83822007000300003&script=sci_arttext

Eamonn, M., et al. (2006). Small intestinal bacterial overgrowth: roles of antibiotics, prebiotics, and probiotics. *Gastroenterology*. 130:578–590. Retrieved from http://www.med.upenn.edu/gastro/documents/Gastroenterologybacterialovergrowth.pdf

Ingram, C. (2008). *The Cure Is in the Cupboard: How to Use Oregano for Better Health*. Vernon Hills, IL: Knowledge House Products.

Laukkarinen, J., et al. (2012). The underlying mechanisms: how hypothyroidism affects the formation of common bile duct stones—a review. *HPB Surgery*. Vol. 2012, 102825. Retrieved from http://dx.doi.org/10.1155/2012/102825

Martin, K. (2007). The chemistry of silica and its potential health benefits. *The Journal of Nutrition Health and Aging*. March-April;11 (2):94-7. Retrieved from http://www.ncbi.nlm.nih.gov/pubmed/17435951

Patrick, L. (2002). Mercury toxicity and antioxidants: Part I: Role of glutathione and alpha-lipoic acid in the treatment of mercury toxicity. *Alternative Medicine Review*, 7(6): 456–471. Retrieved from http://www.altmedrev.com/publications/7/6/456.pdf

Pozzatti, P., et al. (2008). In vitro activity of essential oils extracted from plants used as spices against fluconazole-resistant and fluconazole-susceptible Candida spp. *Canadian Journal of Microbiology*, 54(11):950-956. doi: 10.1139/w08-097. Retrieved from http://www.ncbi.nlm.nih.gov/pubmed/18997851

Shukla, V. & Prakash, A. (1998). Biliary heavy metal concentrations in carcinoma of the gallbladder: case-control study. *British Medical Journal*, 317:1288. doi: 1998;317:1288

Sipos, P., et al. (2003). Some effects of lead contamination on liver and gallbladder bile. *Chemical Research Center, Hungarian Academy of Science, Semmelweis University, Budapest*, 47(1–4):139–142. Retrieved from http://www2.sci.u-szeged.hu/ABS/2003/ActaHP/47139.pdf

Sipos, P., et al. (2003). Some effects of lead contamination on liver and gallbladder bile. *Chemical Research Center, Hungarian Academy of Science, Semmelweis University, Budapest*, 47(1–4):139–142. Retrieved from http://www2.sci.u-szeged.hu/ABS/2003/ActaHP/47139.pdf

Sunĉica D., et. al (2012). Antifungal activity of Oregan (Origanum vulgare L.) extract on the growth of Fusarium and Penicillium species isolated from food. *Scientific Paper*. 66 (1): 33-41. doi: 10.2298/HEMIND110614073K Retrieved from http://www.doiserbia.nb.rs/img/doi/0367-598X/2012/0367-598X1100073K.pdf

Truss, C., et al. (1984). Metabolic abnormalities in patients with chronic candidiasis. The acetaldehyde hypothesis. *Journal of Orthomolecular Psychiatry*. 13(2):66–93. Retrieved from http://www.orthomolecular.org/library/jom/1984/pdf/1984-v13n02-p066.pdf

Uittamo, J., et al. (2009). Chronic candidosis and oral cancer in APECED-patients: Production of carcinogenic acetaldehyde from glucose and ethanol by Candida albicans. *International Journal of Cancer*. 124:754–756. Retrieved from http://onlinelibrary.wiley.com/doi/10.1002/ijc.23976/pdf

Chapter 10: 15 Days of Rest and Recovery

Brownlee, K., Moore, A., & Hackney, A. (2005). Relationship between circulating cortisol and testosterone: influence of physical exercise. *Journal of Sports Science & Medicine* 4(1):76–83. Retrieved from http://www.ncbi.nlm.nih.gov/pubmed/24431964

Georgiou, G. (2007). Body Detox. Retrieved from http://www.collegenatural-medicine.com/images/LBA/body%20detox%202007.pdf

31254484R10065

Made in the USA
San Bernardino, CA
05 March 2016